Checklist
Manual Medicine

Medical Checklists

Series Editors: Alexander Sturm,
Felix Largiadèr, Otto Wicki

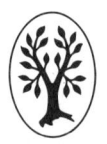

Georg Thieme Verlag Stuttgart · New York
Thieme Medical Publishers, Inc., New York

Checklist
Manual Medicine

Jiří Dvořák, Václav Dvořák
with the cooperation of Hubert Baumgartner
and Ingrid Hannweber

Translated and edited by Wolfgang G. Gilliar

176 illustrations

1991
Georg Thieme Verlag Stuttgart · New York
Thieme Medical Publishers, Inc., New York

Illustrations: Günther Bosch, Stuttgart

Cover design by D. Loenicker, Stuttgart

This book is an authorized translation of the German edition, published and copyrighted 1990 by Georg Thieme Verlag, Stuttgart, Germany.
Title of the German edition: Checkliste Manuelle Medizin.

Die Deutsche Bibliothek — CIP-Einheitsaufnahme

Dvořák, Jiři:
Checklist manual medicine / Jiři Dvořák.
With the cooperation of Hubert Baumgartner and Ingrid Hannweber.
Transl. and ed. by Wolfgang G. Gilliar. [Ill.: Günther Bosch]. –
Stuttgart ; New York : Thieme ; New York : Thieme Med. Publ., 1991
  (Medical checklists)
  Dt. Ausg. u. d. T.: Dvořák, Jiři: Checkliste Manuelle Medizin
NE: Dvořák, Václav;

Important Note: Medicine is an ever-changing science undergoing continual development. Research and clinical experience are continually expanding our knowledge, in particular our knowledge of proper treatment and drug therapy. Insofar as this book mentions any dosage or application, readers may rest assured that the authors, editors and publishers have made every effort to ensure that such references are in accordance with the state of knowledge at the time of production of the book.
Nevertheless this does not involve, imply, or express any guarantee or responsibility on the part of the publishers in respect of any dosage instructions and forms of application stated in the book. Every user is requested to examine carefully the manufacturers' leaflets accompanying each drug and to check, if necessary in consultation with a physician or specialist, whether the dosage schedules mentioned therein or the contraindications stated by the manufacturers differ from the statements made in the present book. Such examination is particularly important with drugs that are either rarely used or have been newly released on the market. Every dosage schedule or every form of application used is entirely at the user's own risk and responsibility. The authors and publishers request every user to report to the publishers any discrepancies or inaccuracies noticed.

Some of the product names, patents and registered designs referred to in this book are in fact registered trademarks or proprietary names even though specific reference to this fact is not always made in the text. Therefore, the appearance of a name without designation as proprietary is not to be construed as a representation by the publisher that it is in the public domain.

This book, including all parts thereof, is legally protected by copyright. Any use, exploitation or commercialization outside the narrow limits set by copyright legislation, without the publisher's consent, is illegal and liable to prosecution. This applies in particular to photostat reproduction, copying, mimeographing or duplication of any kind, translating, preparation of microfilms, and electronic data processing and storage.

© 1991 Georg Thieme Verlag, Rüdigerstraße 14, D-7000 Stuttgart 30, Germany
Thieme Medical Publishers, Inc., 381 Park Avenue South, New York, N.Y. 10016
Typesetting by Robert Hurler GmbH, D-7311 Notzingen (Linotronic 300)
Printed in Germany by Druckhaus Götz KG, D-7140 Ludwigsburg

ISBN 3-13-757701-2 (GTV, Stuttgart)
ISBN 0-86577-386-6 (TMP, New York)   1 2 3 4 5 6

Addresses

Series Editors

Prof. Felix Largiadèr, M.D.,
M.S. (Minn.)
Chairman, Department of
Surgery and Director,
Visceral Surgery Division
University Hospital
Rämistrasse 100
8091 Zürich
Switzerland

Prof. Alexander Sturm, M.D.
Director, Department of
Medicine Hospital
Ruhr University Bochum
Marienhospital
Holkeskampring 40
4690 Herne/Westphalia
Germany

Otto Wicki, M.D.
6707 Iragna
Switzerland

Authors

Jiří Dvořák, M.D.
Head of the Department of
Neurology, Spine Unit
Wilhelm Schulthess Hospital
Neumünsterallee 3
8032 Zürich
Switzerland

Hubert Baumgartner, M.D.
Head of the Department of
Rheumatology, Spine Unit
Wilhelm Schulthess Hospital
Neumünsterallee 10
8032 Zürich
Switzerland

Václav Dvořák, M.D.
Internal and Musculoskeletal
Medicine in General Practice
Dorfstrasse 11
7402 Bonaduz
Switzerland

Ingrid Hannweber
Department of Physiotherapie
Wilhelm Schulthess Hospital
Neumünsterallee 10
8032 Zürich
Switzerland

Translator

Wolfgang G. Gilliar, D.O.
Instructor, Tufts University Medical School,
Dep. of Rehabilitation Medicine
Associate Director, Rehabilitation Medicine,
Greenery Rehabilitation Center
99 Chesnut Hill Ave.
Boston, MA 02135
USA

Series Editors' Preface

The purpose of the Checklist medical series is to present, in a clearly organized manner, up-to-date and field-specific information that serves the reader as both a teaching and reference text. Each book in the series fits into the coat pocket, allowing quick access yet also providing comprehensive information. Dispensing with repetitive material, long indexes, and many cross-references enables this base of knowledge to be presented in such a compact form.

The text at hand has a large target audience. It addresses the practitioner already specialized in manual medicine, as well as many physicians in other specialties, including family practice, orthopedics, surgery, physical medicine and rehabilitation, rheumatology, and last but not least, neurology. The information presented here should also attract the interest of other professionals in the health care system, such as chiropractors and physical therapists.

The addition of this book to the established Checklist series underscores the fact that the field of manual medicine has assumed a solid place in the traditional schools of medicine. This field has already demonstrated its scholarly and scientific methods; the basic principles are comprehensible, learnable, and reproducible.

Several thousand physicians in German-speaking countries have undergone training in this "new" field of medicine. Together they perform a total of about three million manual therapeutic procedures annually. For the first time in such a concentrated form, the great masters in this field, Jiří Dvořák and Václav Dvořák, demonstrate how one acquires knowledge in functional anatomy, how one develops exquisite palpatory skills using one's hands, and how the physician arrives at an active diagnosis, so as to finally apply the appropriate therapeutic technique or method. The goal is to ameliorate the patient's pain and discomfort.

We, the editors of this series, would like to extend our thanks to the doctors Dvořák for their collegial and harmonic cooperation and for their compliance with our requests for keeping the information about the various components of manual medicine as brief as possible without sacrificing substance. We anticipate that this book will find a large number of interested readers.

Iragna, Zurich, Herne-Bochum

Otto Wicki
Felix Largiadèr
Alexander Sturm

Authors' Preface

A recent survey conducted by the Swiss Association of Resident and Senior Physicians (VSAO) and a survey of practicing physicians in the Swiss canton of Bern indicate that there is a great demand for further education in manual medicine by young physicians as well as those already established in their practice.

More than 90% of the physicians surveyed would utilize manual medicine techniques when indicated, and up to 75% of the physicians would like to receive competent training in this field. These figures are impressive, as they document the vastly growing interest in this field among young physicians.

In a few European countries, such as Austria, France, Denmark, and Germany, manual medicine has gained entrance to the universities, albeit to a rather modest extent. In Switzerland as well, lectures have been presented to students as an introduction to the field. The cautious acceptance of manual medicine by the traditional medical faculties is understandable and, yes, undoubtedly justified; for a long time, practitioners of manual medicine and chiropractors had used terminology with which the traditional fields of medicine had not been familiar. As long as the principles of a new method cannot be explained in an understandable language, the proponents of such a method cannot expect to be welcomed with open arms into the traditional schools. Each treatment method that bases its therapeutic success on empirical experience is required to subject itself to scientifically accepted methodology and standards.

In the text at hand we have integrated such fundamental elements as basic biomechanics and functional anatomy of the musculoskeletal system, as well as simple and reproducible examination techniques and practical treatment procedures. It is our intention to stimulate interest and provide an introduction to manual medicine for both the medical student and the practicing physician. We would be delighted if this introduction were to become the source of motivation for further education in this field.

This book is primarily based on topics covered in two standard texts on manual medicine published by Thieme, namely *Manual Medicine: Diagnostics*, 2nd ed. (J. Dvořák and V. Dvořák, 1990), and *Manual Medicine: Therapy* (W. Schneider, J. Dvořák, V. Dvořák, T. Tritschler, 1988). As editors of these two volumes, we were especially pleased when we were asked to put together this text for the Checklist series. We know that, due to its high quality, the Checklist series is held in high esteem among medical professionals.

We would like to thank the physicians team of the Wilhelm Schulthess Hospital, especially Prof. N. Gschwend, Prof. H. Scheier, Dr. H. Baumgartner, Dr. U. Munzinger, Dr. D. Grob, and Dr. B. Simmen. They made it possible for manual medicine to become a logical component of treatment within the concepts of orthopedics and rheumatology. It is in the interdisciplinary clinic meetings, where the orthopedist, rheumatologist, neurologist, and manual medicine practitioner come together, that not only the limits but also the advantages of new treatment approaches become apparent. In the functional assessment of a patient with musculoskeletal problems, it is important to know when and for how long the patient would benefit from a rational conservative approach before it becomes a wasteful intervention or even a negative one.

We would also like to extend our sincere appreciation to Judith Reichert, who not only revised the text, but demonstrated the outstanding graphic capabilities of desktop publishing; also Christiana Vincenz has been very helpful in putting the manuscript together.

Furthermore, and with great gratitude, we would like to thank the editors of the Checklist series, Prof. F. Largiadèr, Dr. O. Wicki, and Prof. A. Sturm, as well as Dr. Bremkamp of Thieme Publishers, for their support and realization of this project.

Zurich and Bonaduz, April 1991   Jiří Dvořák
Václav Dvořák

Contents

Functional Anatomy 1
Biomechanics 1
   Neurophysiology of the Joints 22

Manual Diagnosis 26
Functional Examination 26
   Concepts of Manual Diagnosis 26

Examination Techniques 30
Cervical Spine 30
Cervical Spine − Cervicothoracic Junction 34
Cervical Spine 39
Cervical Spine − Cervicothoracic Junction 42
Cervical Spine 45
Thoracic Spine 46
Rib I 49
Ribs III to XII 50
Lumbar Spine 51
Lower Lumbar Spine 55
Pelvic Girdle 56
Shoulder Girdle 60
Elbow 66
Hand 69
Knee Joints 74
Foot 78
Pectoralis major Muscle 83
Trapezius Muscle 84
Levator scapulae Muscle 86
Sternocleidomastoid Muscle 88
Scalene Muscles 90
Erector spinae Muscle, Longissimus lumborum Muscle 92
Piriform Muscle 94
Psoas major Muscle 96
Rectus femoris Muscle 98
Hamstring Muscles 100
Abdominal Muscles 102
Gluteus maximus Muscle 104
Gluteus medius Muscle 105
Cervical Spine 106
Thoracic Spine 110
Lumbar Spine 113
Sacroiliac Joint and Pelvis 115

Radiologic Diagnosis 117
   Cervical Spine 117
   Thoracic Spine 119
   Lumbar Spine and Pelvis 121

Indications, Contraindications, Complications 128
Indications 128
Contraindications 130

Manual Therapy 131
Concepts of Manual Therapy 131
  Basic Principles 132
Cervical Spine 138
Cervicothoracic Junction 146
Thoracic Spine 148
Ribs 152
Lumbar Spine 155
Sacroiliac Joint 161
Pectoralis major Muscles 166
Trapezius Muscle, Descending Portion 167
Levator scapulae Muscle 168
Sternocleidomastoid Muscle 169
Iliopsoas Muscle 170
Rectus femoris Muscle 171
Piriformis Muscle 172
Biceps femoris Muscle, Semitendinosus Muscle,
Semimembranosus Muscle 173

Back School 174

Index 179

Functional Anatomy
Biomechanics

Functional Anatomy

- The analysis of normal and abnormal movement requires a well-founded knowledge of functional anatomy.
- A functional disturbance of the paravertebral muscles and deep back muscles will lead to abnormal movement or will alter movement sequence. When muscles become shortened, actual motion restriction may be present.
- True paralysis of the paravertebral muscles, e. g. as with poliomyelitis, will inevitably elicit abnormal postural relationships among the various spinal regions, such as progressive scoliosis and kyphosis.
- Symmetrical contraction of the short and long paravertebral muscles is accompanied by extension of the spine.
- Rotation of the head and trunk to one side is induced by the ipsilateral long back extensors, the abdominal muscles, as well as the contralateral small muscles of the transversospinal system, namely the semispinal muscle, the multifidus muscle and the rotator muscles (Fig. **1**).

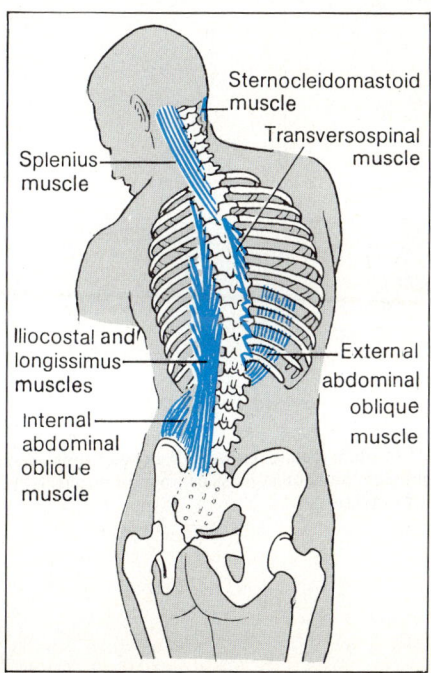

Fig. 1 Anatomic diagram: rotation of the trunk to the left and the associated contracted muscles (after Rickenbacher et al., 1982)

Functional Anatomy
Biomechanics

- Range of motion between the individual spinal segments is controlled by the ipsilateral transversospinal system, while regional control is achieved by the contralateral long back extensors (Fig. 2).
- During side-bending movement, which is always coupled with rotation movement, both the ipsilateral and contralateral muscles work together in a coordinated fashion.

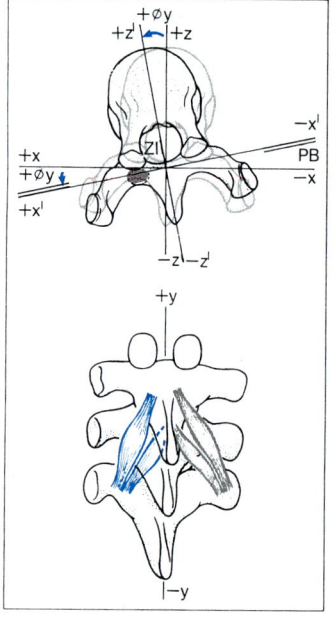

Fig. 2 Conflict situation (present resting position). Dark blue: shortened agonist muscles (rotators). Light blue: antagonist muscles (rotator muscles). PB: pathologic barrier. ZI: zone of irritation
$+z-(+z') = +\emptyset y \frown$
$+x-(+x') = +\emptyset y \frown$

Functional Anatomy
Biomechanics

- The rich supply of muscle spindles in the small transversospinal muscles emphasizes their importance in the control and regulation of both segmental and regional (i.e., gross) movement.
- Upright body posture relies on the interplay of the straight and oblique abdominal muscles and the long back extensors.
- Functional weakness or organic paresis/paralysis of the abdominal muscles is associated with a decrease in intra-abdominal pressure which then may lead to an exaggerated lumbar lordosis.
- Thus, the intervertebral disks as well as the apophyseal (facet) joints become susceptible and vulnerable to undue stress and overload.

Functional Pathology of Muscle

- Human skeletal muscle is comprised of thousands of muscle fibers. A single muscle fiber is about as thin as a hair and can reach a length of 10−15 cm.
- In general, a distinction is made between two types of muscle fibers: the type-I fibers, the so-called slow twitch fibers, and the type-II fibers, the fast twitch fibers.
- The postural (tonic) muscles have a significantly higher proportion of slow twitch fibers, whereas the phasic muscles are composed primarily of fast twitch fibers.
- The primary function of the tonic muscles (postural muscles) is to maintain upright posture. For energy supply, they predominately rely on the aerobic mechanism, and the primary energy source is glycogen and fat. Production of lactic acid is rather small.
- The phasic muscles can undergo the most rapid (fast twitch) contractions, receiving their energy from glycogen in the anaerobic cycle with rapid accumulation of lactic acid.
- Capillary supply to the slow twitch fibers is notably higher than that to the fast twitch fibers. Thus, the slow twitch fibers do not fatigue until after several hundred contractions. In constrast, the fast twitch fibers fatigue very rapidly, often after only a few contractions (Table **1**).

Functional Anatomy
Biomechanics

Table 1 Characteristics of slow twitch and fast twitch muscle fibers

Flexion	Slow Twitch (I)	Fast Twitch (II)
Function	tonic (postural)	phasic
Twitch speed	slow	fast
Metabolism/enzymes	oxidative	glycolytic
Myosin ATPase	low activity	high activity
Fatigability rate	slow	rapid
"Color"	red	white
Capillary density	high	low
Spindle number	high	moderate
Innervation	α_2-motor neuron	α_1-motor neuron
Reaction to functional disturbance	shortening	weakening

- In the presence of a functional disturbance, the postural muscles tend to shorten, whereas the phasic muscles responsible for rapid movements tend to become weak. This disrupts the balanced interplay of muscle action, leading to muscular imbalance (Janda, 1979). As a result, normal physiologic movement and movement sequences (movement patterns) are altered, affecting the various spinal regions and/or extremity joints.
- Table 2 and Figure 3 review the important postural and phasic muscles.

Myotendinosis

- The healthy muscle displays normal plasticity and uniform consistency; the individual muscle bundles cannot be differentiated from each other by palpation.
- Myotendinotic changes are characterized by increased tone, greater palpatory resistance and decreased suppleness. When palpating perpendicularly to the muscle fiber direction, only minimal to moderate pressure is necessary to elicit pain in an affected muscle portion. This allows differentiation from the unaffected remainder of the muscle. Myotendinosis can be palpated from the origin to the insertion of the muscle. "Nervous misinformation" from certain muscle portions, mediated through reflex pathways, is responsible for the involuntary isometric increase in tone in the muscle bundle (Fig. 4).

Functional Anatomy
Biomechanics

Table 2 Overview of the important muscles with primarily phasic or tonic function (adapted from Janda, 1979).

Primarily postural (tonic) muscles	Primarily phasic muscles
Trunk	
Erector spinae muscles in lumbar and cervical region	Erector spinae muscles in mid-thoracic region
Quadratus lumborum	
Scalene muscles	
Shoulder Girdle	
Pectoralis major	Rhomboid muscles
Levator scapulae	Trapezius (ascending)
Trapezius (descending portion)	Trapezius (horizontal)
Biceps brachii (short head)	Pectoralis (abdominal)
Biceps brachii (long head)	Triceps brachii
Pelvic Region/Thigh	
Biceps femoris	Vastus medialis
Semitendinosus	Vastus lateralis
Semimembranosus	
Iliopsoas	Gluteus medius
Rectus femoris	Gluteus maximus
	Gluteus minimus
Tensor fasciale latae	
Adductor longus	
Adductor brevis	
Adductor magnus	
Gracilis	
Piriformis	
Calf and Foot	
Gastrocnemius	Tibialis anterior
Soleus	Peroneal muscles

Functional Anatomy
Biomechanics

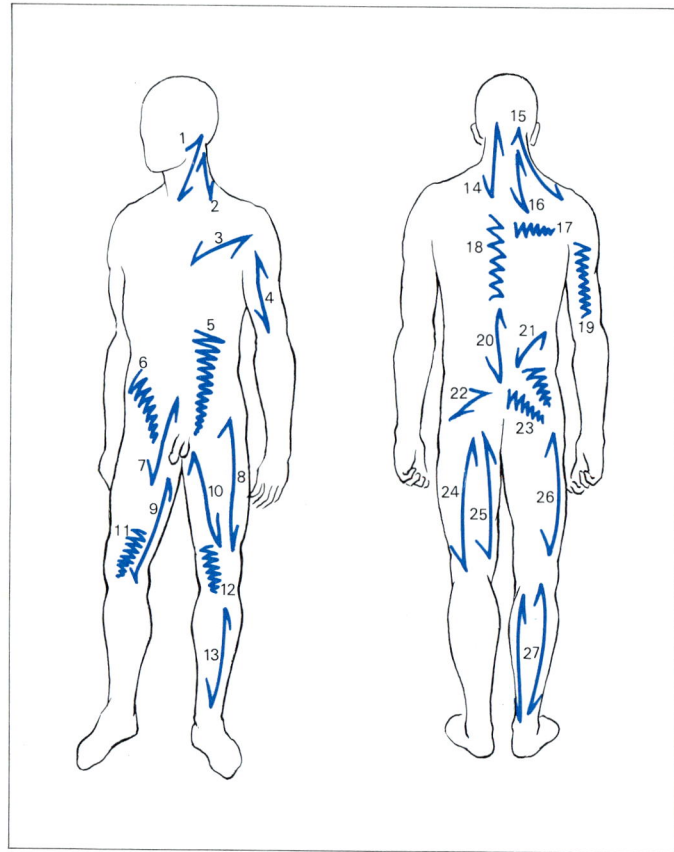

Fig. 3 Overview of the postural (⇀) and phasic (〰) muscles
 1 Sternocleidomastoid muscle
 2 Scalene muscles
 3 Pectoralis major muscle
 4 Biceps brachii muscle
 5 Rectus abdominis muscle
 6 Abdominal oblique muscle
 7 Iliopsoas muscle
 8 Rectus femoris muscle
 9 Gracilis muscle
10 Adductors
11 Vastus medialis muscle
12 Vastus lateralis muscle
13 Tibialis anterior muscle
14 Longissimus cervicis muscle
15 Trapezius muscle (descending portion)
16 Levator scapulae muscle
17 Rhomboid muscles
18 Longissimus dorsi muscle
19 Triceps brachii muscle
20 Longissimus dorsi muscle
21 Quadratus lumborum muscle
22 Piriform muscle
23 Gluteal muscles
24 Biceps femoris muscle
25 Semitendinosus muscle
26 Tensor fasciae latae muscle
27 Triceps surae muscle
    (soleus and gatrocnemius muscles)

Functional Anatomy
Biomechanics

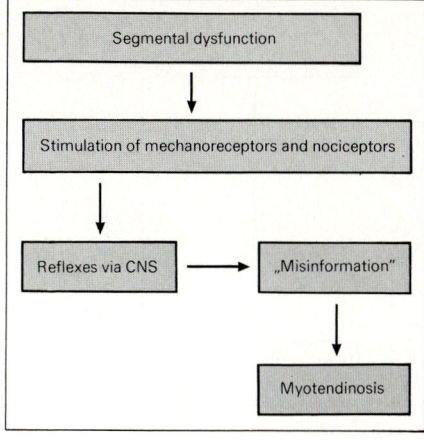

Fig. 4 Development of myotendinosis (after Fassbender, 1980)

Myosis

- Continuous increased muscle tone (taut, palpable band) will, after a certain latency period, lead to myosis in the muscle and to tendinosis in the inserting tendon. This is known in the rheumatological literature as noninflammatory soft-tissue rheumatism (Fig. 5).
- Myosis is described as altered (increased) muscle tissue texture, which is painful upon palpatory pressure or spontaneously. Myoses are found primarily in the center of the muscle mass. Particularly frequently they are found at sites where the muscle changes direction or at the free muscle borders (e. g., trapezius muscle, pectoralis major muscle).

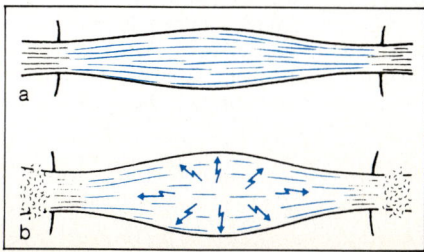

Fig. 5 a Normal muscle. b Tendomyotically altered muscle (schematic)

Functional Anatomy
Biomechanics

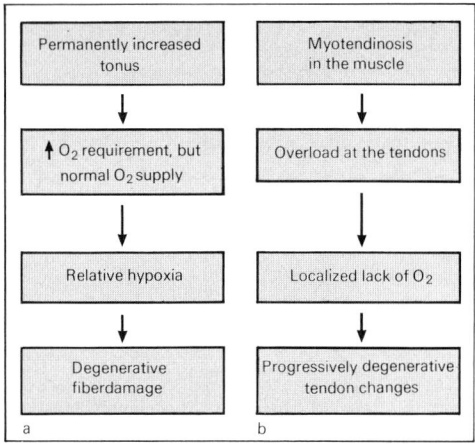

Fig. 6 Pathology of noninflammatory soft-tissue rheumatism (after Fassbender, 1980). **a** Muscle myosis. **b** Tendinosis (ligaments and tendon)

- Continued nonphysiologic irritation and constantly increased tone is accompanied by degenerative changes, resulting in muscle fiber damage (Fig. **6**). So-called attachment tendinoses are well-localized swellings of tendons, confined to their respective origins and insertions. These become extremely painful upon palpation. Characteristically they present symmetrically, like mirror images. In addition to the typical sites of origin and insertion, tendinoses can appear just as well at the muscle−tendon junction and are named transition tendinoses.
- Due to the reflexes involved, tendinoses and myoses become apparent not immediately, but rather after a certain delay. By the same token, they do not disappear immediately with the correction of the original disturbance but rather after a certain delay. This important finding helps to diagnostically distinguish the entities just described from the zones of irritation (described below).
- A certain muscle contains the same amount of defined longitudinal sections that, independently from each other but in a set sequence, can undergo tone changes (hard, palpable bands). Such a clinical "muscle unit" and its associated tendons have been named a myotenone.

Functional Anatomy
Biomechanics

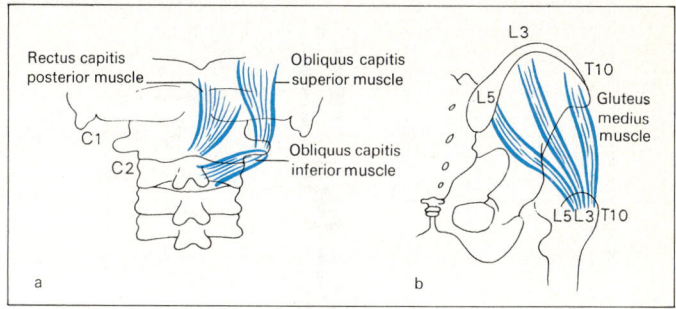

Fig. 7 **a** Individual myotenones. **b** Myotenones in a fan-shaped muscle

- A single myotenone consists of a narrow muscle, whereas broad, flat, and fan-shaped muscles comprise several myotenones (Fig. **7**).
- Clinical experience has shown that specific axial skeletal parts can be correlated with certain myotenones, clinical findings that can be reproduced symmetrically, qualitatively, and objectively.
- The primary spondylogenic pain syndrome is that in which there is a primary functional disturbance/position in a spinal segment (i.e. segmental somatic dysfunction), accompanied by increased muscle tone (taut, palpable band) and the formation of myotendinoses.

Biomechanics

- Any movement in space can be defined within the framework of a three-dimensional coordinate system. Derived from general principles in the field of mechanics, this system has also found general acceptance and application in biomechanics, allowing precise definition of movement and movement patterns. Three primary axes are utilized in this coordinate system (Fig. **8**):
-   – the transverse, horizontal x-axis,
    – the vertical y-axis, and
    – the sagittal z-axis.
- The combination of two of the three axes defines the three major planes in this coordinate system. This allows analysis of each individual motion component in reference to these axes and planes, or practically, according to the rotation about a specific axis in a specific plane. Rotation is defined with respect to the axis involved.
-   – Flexion and extension: rotation about the x-axis
    – Side-bending: rotation about the z-axis
    – Axial rotation: rotation about the y-axis (Fig. **8**)

Functional Anatomy
Biomechanics

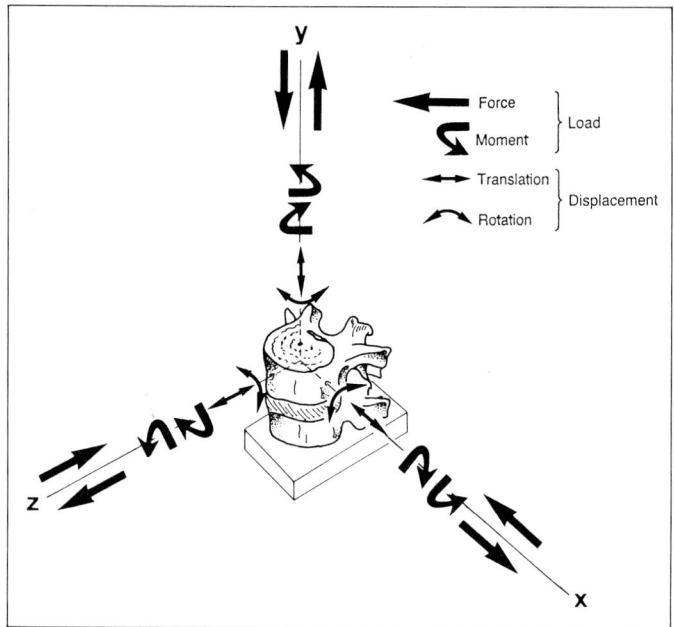

Fig. 8 A three-dimensional coordinate system has been placed at the center of the upper vertebral body of a vertebral unit (motion segment). A total of 12 load components, linear and rotatory, can act on these axes; the application of any one of the load components (linear or rotatory) produces displacement of the upper vertebra with respect to the lower vertebra. This displacement consists of translation and rotation (after White and Panjabi, 1990)

- When interpreting either gross movement of the spine or specific segmental movement, the following conventional rules are kept in mind: When describing rotation about a particular axis, the point of reference is the superior and anterior aspect of the vertebral body in question (Fig. **9**).
- Movement between two adjacent vertebrae (the two partners of a spinal segment), is defined as that of the superior vertebra in relationship to its inferior partner.
- Axial rotation and side-bending in an individual spinal segment are coupled with each other, for which the term "coupling pattern" has been coined.

Functional Anatomy
Biomechanics

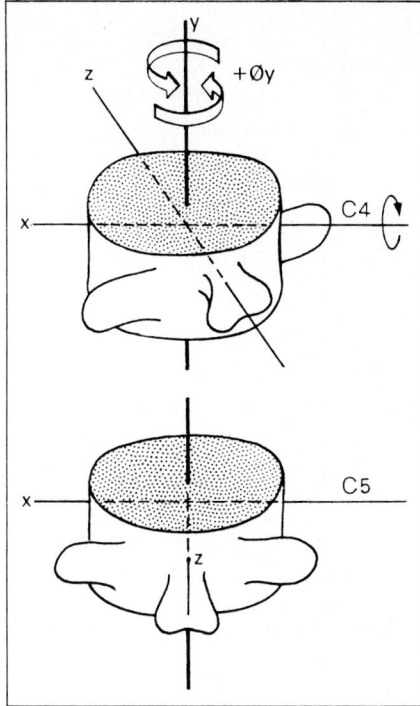

Fig. 9 Definition of rotation movement

Upper Cervical Spine (Fig. 10)

- Occiput—C0, Atlas—C1, Axis—C2.
- Atlanto-occipital joints: Range of motion for flexion/extension = 8–13°, with limitation due to the bony structures and surrounding soft tissues (Note: Inclination and reclination movement were specifically termed to denote flexion and extension in the cervical spinal area, respectively).
- Side-bending measures 4° to either side and is greatest when the head is slightly flexed.
- During side-bending, a coupled rotation to the same side (forced rotation) occurs in the second vertebra and the one below. The axis is able rotate more during maximal side-bending than with maximal rotation of the cervical spine (forced rotation of the axis).

Functional Anatomy
Biomechanics

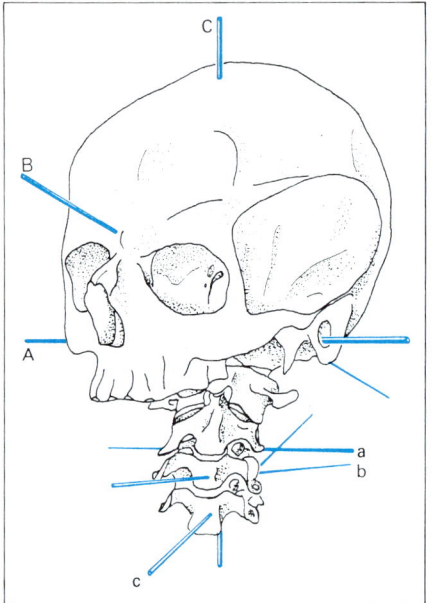

Fig. **10** Axes of motion of the occipital-atlanto-axial and cervical joints (after Knese, 1947/50); A = transverse axis for flexion in upper cervical joints; B = sagittal axis for side-bending in upper cervical joints; C = rotational axis; a = transverse axis of the lower cervical joints; b = axis for side-bending in lower cervical joints; c = axis for side-bending of the cervical spine

- In the upper cervical spine, the atlas undergoes a lateral displacement in the direction of the side-bending, as well as an axis rotation. This can be visualized in the AP radiograph of the cervical spine when there is an asymmetry in the distance between the dens of the axis and either lateral mass of the atlas (Fig. **11**).
- In the atlanto-occipital joints, rotation of about 4° can take place, but may actually become significantly increased when there is atlantoaxial arthrosis or fusion of the atlanto-occipital joints.
- The atlantoaxial articulations consist of 4 joint spaces, one of which has been described as a bursa: this is the space between the transverse ligament of the atlas and the dens of the axis.

Functional Anatomy
Biomechanics

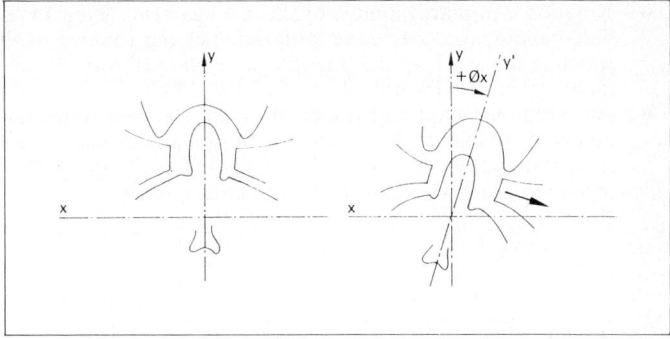

Fig. 11 Gliding movement of the atlas with side-bending to the right

- The joint surfaces between C1 and C2 are convex. Laterally, a wedgelike synovial fold takes up the space of the otherwise rather flabby and fibrous joint capsule (meniscoid) (Fig. **12**).
- The primary movement in the lower cervical spine is axial rotation, which in healthy adolescents measures approximately 43° to either side. This constitutes approximately half of the entire cervical spine rotation.

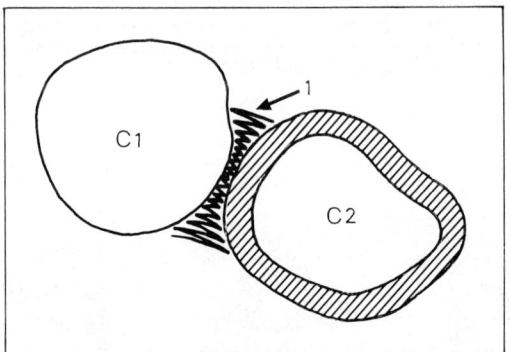

Fig. 12 The exposed atlantoaxial joint after transecting through the flabby fibrous joint capsule. The hatched area indicates the location of the wedgelike synovial fold (meniscoid), the functional of which is to balance the gapping in the atlantoaxial joint. 1) joint capsule; 2) position of the meniscoid (after Dvorak, 1988)

Functional Anatomy
Biomechanics

- Rotation is primarily limited by the alar ligaments (Figs. **13** and **14**). Side-bending can only occur with simultaneous rotation of the axis which is the result of the physiologic relationships of the alar ligaments (Fig. **15**) (Dvořák, J. et al., 1987, 1988).
- An additional important function of the alar and transverse ligaments of the atlas is that of limiting flexion and extension as well as axial rotation. Both of these ligaments are made up mostly of collagenous fibers which allow only minimal stretch.

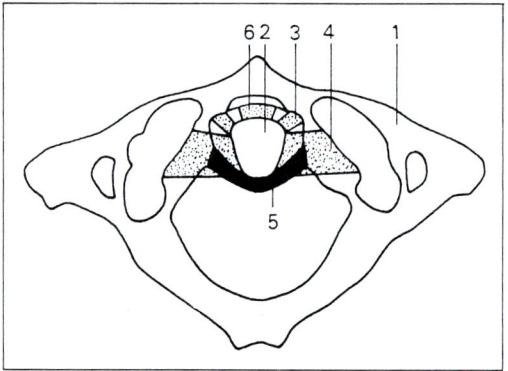

Fig. **13** Schematic representation of the ligamentous apparatus at the craniocervical junction. 1) atlas; 2) dens of the axis; 3) atlantal portion of the alar ligament; 4) occipital portion of the alar ligament; 5) transverse ligament of the atlas; 6) anterior atlantodental ligament

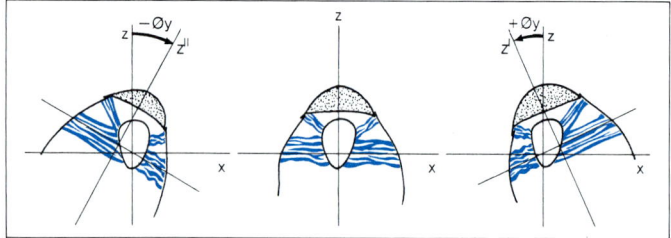

Fig. **14** Function of the alar ligaments during rotation in the atlantoaxial joint (C1–C2):
z–z' rotation to the right; z–z'' rotation to the left

Functional Anatomy
Biomechanics

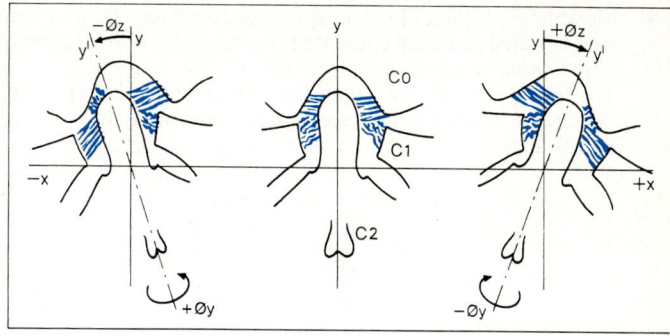

Fig. 15 Function of the alar ligaments during side-bending in the atlantoaxial joint (C1–C2)

- During atlantoaxial rotation to one side, the opposite ligament will become taut, thus limiting movement. In side-bending, however, it is the ipsilateral ligament that becomes tight during the first phase. During the second phase, the atlantodental connection, which is felt to be an integral part of the alar ligament, will also become tight, preventing further displacement of the atlas in direction of side-bending (Fig. **15**).

Midcervical and Lower Cervical Spine (C3–C7)

- The axis can be viewed as a transitional vertebra between the upper and lower cervical spine. Greatest range of movement occurs in the midcervical spine, where the following movements are possible: flexion and extension, side-bending, and rotation.
- The inclination of the facets in the midcervical and lower cervical spine measures 45° to the horizontal plane (Fig. **16**).

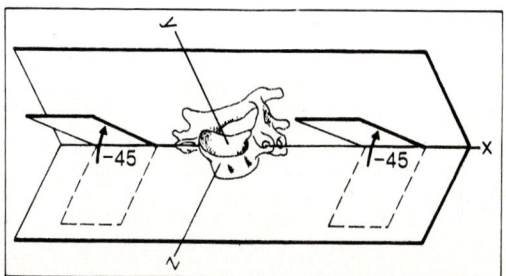

Fig. 16 Facet joint inclinations and axes of motion for vertebra C4 (after White and Panjabi, 1990)

15

Functional Anatomy
Biomechanics

- Movement in the individual spinal segments occurs as a combination of translatory and rotatory movement about the respective axis in the three-dimensional coordinate system.
- The top angle of the individual spinal segments is determined by the inclination of the joint surfaces and the funtion of the intervertebral disc (Fig. **17**).

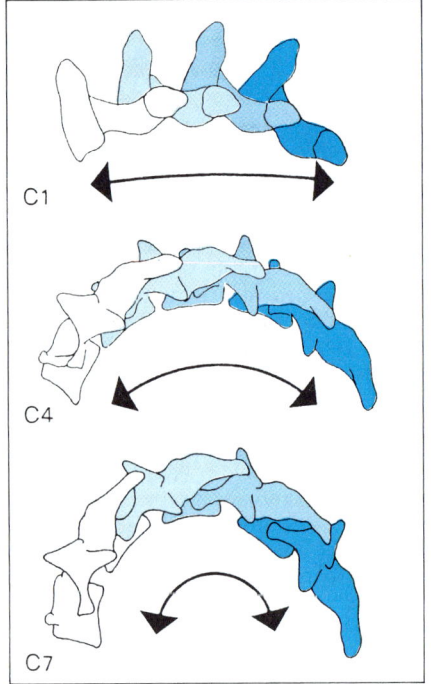

Fig. **17** The segmental arches (after Lysell, 1969)

- The greatest extent of flexion and extension occurs in the midcervical spinal segments. The greatest range of motion is measured at the spinal segment C5−C6, measuring on average 24°. This fact has often been linked to the increased incidence of cervical spondyloarthrosis and osteochondrosis in the mid portion of the cervical spine.
- Translatory gliding in the sagittal plane ($\pm$ z-axis) measures approximately 2−3.5 mm.

Functional Anatomy
Biomechanics

Vertebral Artery

- The vertebral artery enters the costotransverse foramen of C6, rarely that of C5, and runs up to the axis through the transverse foramina of the individual vertebrae. It enters the costotransverse foramen of the atlas and upon its exit forms a posterosuperiorly directed loop.
- Extreme head rotation can lead to dizziness, nausea, tinnitus, etc. This may be due to a transient decrease in blood supply in the basilar region.
- Rotation of the head between 30° and 45° to one side causes the blood flow to be diminished in the opposite vertebral artery at the level of the atlantoaxial junction (Fig. **18**).

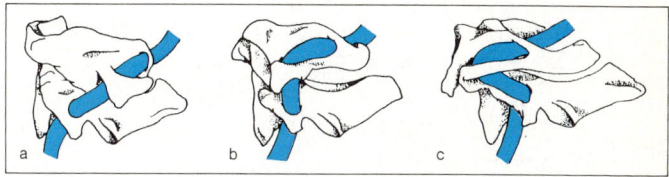

Fig. **18a–c** Course of the left vertebral artery during atlas rotation to the left and right (after Fielding, 1957)

- A constitutional or acquired posttraumatic rotation instability of the upper cervical spine can lead to mechanical reduction of blood flow. The close topographical proximity of the vertebral artery with the margins of the C1–C2 joints during axial rotation may also allow reflex spasms of the vertebral artery due to mechanical irritation.
- These considerations are to be kept in mind when manipulating the cervical spine (classical thrust techniques or mobilization with impulse techniques), so as to prevent any adverse effects.
- *Reclination test:* With the patient sitting, the examiner introduces movement of the head to either side, starting from the neutral and extension position. These passive movements should be performed very slowly and the patient should immediately report any symptoms (subjective findings).

Functional Anatomy
Biomechanics

- *De Kleijn hanging test:* The patient is supine, and the examiner holds the patient's head beyound the examination table. From this hanging position the head is passively rotated to either side. The appearance of nystagmus and/or subjective symptoms is looked for.

Thoracic Spine

- At the cervicothoracic junction, the inclination of the joint surface is more vertical, with rotation about the x-axis measuring 60° and about the y-axis measuring 20° (Fig. **19**).

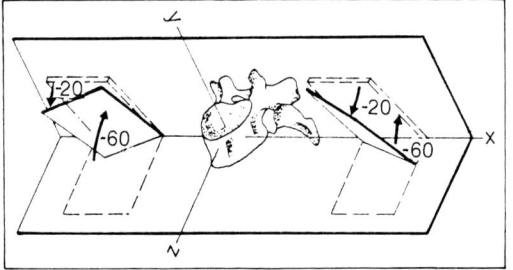

Fig. 19 The facet joint inclinations and axes of motion of a thoracic vertebra (after White and Panjabi, 1990)

- Due to this double inclination of the facet joint surfaces and the anterior connection of the individual thoracic vertebrae with the ribs and the sternum, only minimal segmental mobility can take place.
- Starting from the midthoracic spine, flexion and extension movement increase in range of motion.
- Side-bending is always coupled with rotation towards the same side. Clinically, the spinous processes move towards the convexity that is in a direction opposite that of the side-bending (Fig. **20**).

Lumbar Spine

- The joint surfaces of the lumbar spinal facet joints are almost vertical and rotated approximately 45° about the y-axis (Fig. **21**).
- This rather vertical orientation prevents axial rotation in particular. In the spinal segment L5−S1, rotation of only 5° is possible.
- The primary movement in the lumbar spine is flexion and extension.

Functional Anatomy
Biomechanics

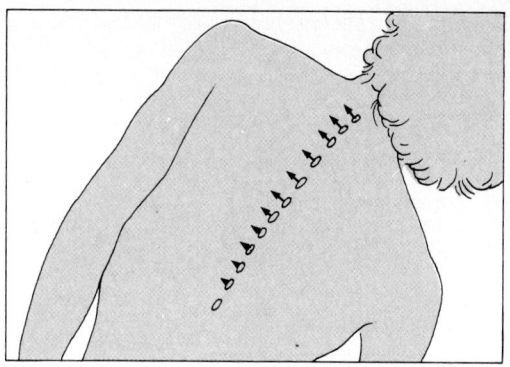

Fig. 20 Gross motion testing of side-bending movement

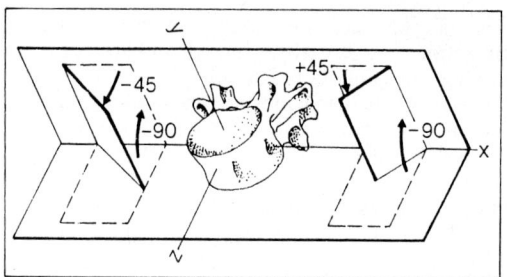

Fig. 21 The facet joint inclinations and axes of motion of a lumbar vertebra (after White and Panjabi, 1990)

Pelvic Girdle

- The functional unit of the pelvic girdle consists of the sacrum, both ilia, the 5th lumbar vertebra connected through the sacroiliac joints on either side, and the symphysis pubis anteriorly.
- Structurally these sacroiliac joints are a diarthrosis, but due to the anatomic orientation of the joint surface, they function more as an amphiarthrosis.
- The sacroiliac joint assumes a C shape (Fig. 22), and the joint surfaces are covered by cartilage.

Functional Anatomy
Biomechanics

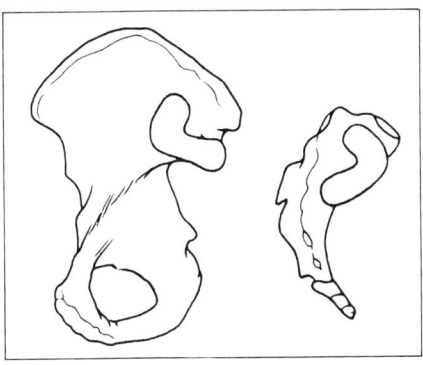

Fig. 22 Anatomic arrangement of the sacroiliac joint

- The cartilage of the sacroiliac joints undergoes degenerative changes rather soon, and as early as the 4th and 5th decades of life, erosions may become apparent. Already in the 6th decade, bony bridging as well as neoarthrosis may be observed, as may complete ankylosis.
- The interosseous sacroiliac ligament is very important as it guarantees the interlocking between the sacrum and both ilia, not unlike the function of a suspension bridge (Fig. 23).

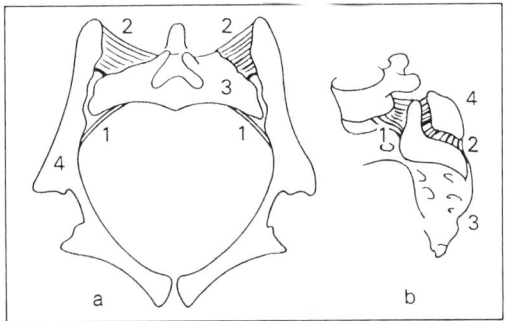

Fig. 23 The sacral suspension (schematic), superior view (**a**; after Kapandji, 1974) and medial view (**b**). 1) anterior sacroiliac ligament; 2) interosseous sacroiliac ligament; 3) sacrum; 4) ilium

Functional Anatomy
Biomechanics

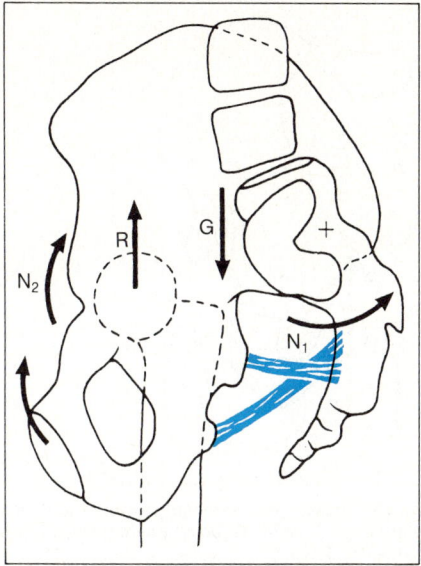

Fig. 24 Body posture and its effects on the sacroiliac joint (after Kapandji, 1974). G: body weight (gravity); R: reaction of the ground; N1: nutation motion of sacrum; N2: counternutation by the innominate bone

- Rotational movement of the sacrum between the ilia has been termed "nutation" (nodding) movement. During both standing and the gait cycle, tremendous forces act on the sacroiliac joints (Fig. **24**).
- During the gait cycle, various force relationships apply so as to alternatingly allow physiologic intrapelvic distortions or reversible pelvic torsions.
- Nutation movement of the sacrum and counternutation of the iliac bone during gait is enhanced by the active contraction of the hamstring muscles, as well as the gluteus maximus, iliopsoas, and quadriceps femoris muscles.
- Standing on one leg causes the opposite sacroiliac joint to undergo nutation movement while the ipsilateral symphysis moves inferiorly (Fig. **25**).

Functional Anatomy
Biomechanics

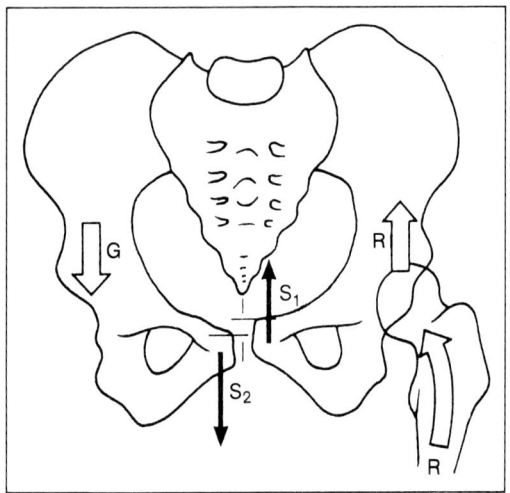

Fig. 25 Shearing forces encountered at the symphysis during stance phase (standing on one leg; after Kapandji, 1974). G: body weight (gravity); R: reaction of the ground; S1, S2: shearing forces

Neurophysiology of the Joints

- The intervertebral joints are diarthroses, as are the uncovertebral joints in the cervical spine.
- The articular surfaces are covered by cartilage, the joint capsules contain synovia and, depending on the vertebral region, they have very strong collagenous fibers.
- The meniscoids or invaginations of the synovial fold smoothen irregularities of the joint surfaces, in particular at the cervical spine. These are vascularized and innervated (Fig. 26).
- The fibrous joint capsules reveal mechanoreceptors as well as nociceptive free nerve endings (nociceptors).
- Tension and stretching of the joint capsule is monitored through the mechanoreceptors. Changes in tension and pressure will reflexly alter not only the paravertebral muscular tone, but also muscles in the extremities.
- The free, very small, myelinated plexiform nerve endings (nociceptors) may become depolarized as a result of constant pressure upon the joint capsule (nonphysiologic position, abnormally quick movement), as well as a result of a decrease in the intervertebral disk height and dislocated of the facet joints. Chemical irritation due to

Functional Anatomy
Biomechanics

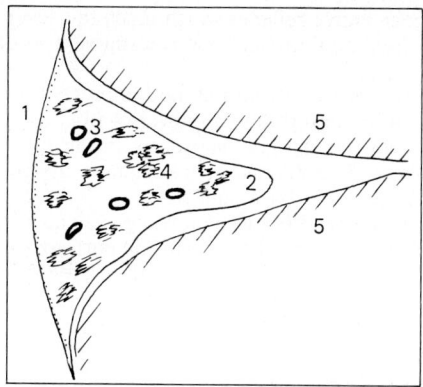

Fig. 26 Meniscoid (schematic representation). 1) joint capsule; 2) meniscoid; 3) blood vessels; 4) fatty tissue; 5) articular surfaces (facet joint)

K^+ ions 5-hydroxytryptamine, and histamines may also lead to depolarization of the free nerve endings, which in turn leads to pain.
- The joint capsules are innervated by the dorsal rami of the spinal nerves. However, one particular ramus is not responsible for only one segmentally related joint capsule but sends out lateral branches connecting to the neighboring proximal and distal apophyseal (facet) joints as well.
- This plurisegmental innervation of the facet joints is of significant importance for the coordination of complex regional movement patterns. This may also explain the fact that the pain described by the patient often cannot be localized to one segment as it is perceived over an area covering several segments (overlap of the dermatomas).
- The small myelinated nociceptive fibers, as well as the fast fibers conducting information from the mechanoreceptors, enter through the posterior portion of the dorsal root reaching the dorsal horn of the gray substance in the spinal cord.
- The nociceptive fibers connect with the basal nuclei, and via the spinothalamic tract, the information is transmitted to the limbic system, where actual pain perception occurs.
- The afferent information from the mechanoreceptors is also transmitted through the dorsal roots to the dorsal horn. Parts of the fibers connect with the basal nuclei through inhibitory interneurons.

Functional Anatomy
Biomechanics

- The pain-inducing nociceptive reflexes which reach this level are in part presynaptically inhibited, interrupting transmission to the spinothalamic tract.
- The majority of the information from the mechanoreceptors, however, is transmitted to the brainstem via posterior fibers.
- The substantia gelatinosa of the gray substance in the spinal cord produces its own opiates. The increase in enkephalins interrupts the nociceptive transmission in the basal nuclei.
- Strong stimulation of the type-II mechanoreceptors causes an increase of enkephalins in the dorsal horns. This, in part, may explain the positive pain-reducing effect seen with passive physical therapeutic measure, including manual therapy.
- Figures **27** and **28** delineate possible mechanisms involved in the development of segmental and regional dysfunction as well as the influences of specific manipulative therapy.

Functional Anatomy
Biomechanics

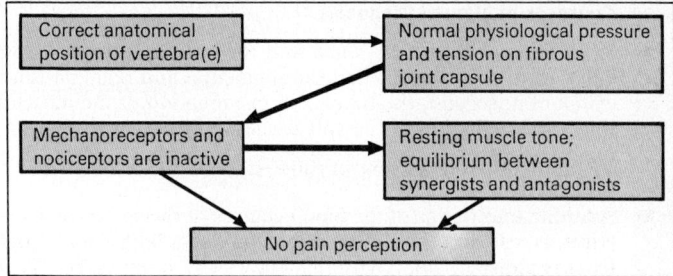

Fig. 27 Model for receptor activity when vertebrae are in the correct position

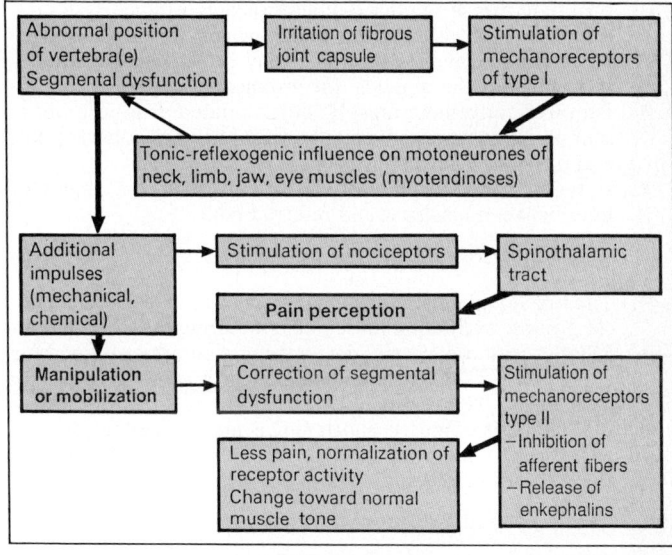

Fig. 28 Model for receptor activity when vertebrae are in an abnormal position (segmental dysfunction)

Manual Diagnosis
Functional Examination

Concepts of Manual Diagnosis

- The examination of the spine and the extremity joints can be divided into three steps: First, the segmental and regional functional evaluation; second, the functional examination of the muscles; and third, the palpation of the soft tissues.

Functional Examination of the Spine

- A Sound knowledge of the biomechanics of the spine and its related joints as well as a three-dimensional understanding of the joint surfaces is indispensable. With this knowledge in mind, one is able to perform a more detailed regional examination, comparing the range of motion in a particular region of the spine, both actively and passively.
- Range of motion is measured in degrees of rotation about the appropriate axis in the three-dimensional coordinate system. In addition, one also evaluates the endfeel which appears hard when there are articular changes or which may be soft-elastic when there is shortening of the muscles, for instance.
- Pain with movement must be differentiated as to whether it is present at the onset of movement or if it becomes apparent only at the end of passive movement.
- In regard to the location of the patient's pain, one should differentiate between localized and referred pain.

Functional Examination of the Muscles

- The functional muscle examination concentrates on individual muscle groups, evaluating muscle length, strength, and endurance.
- Muscles with a primarily postural function are examined for shortening, whereas the phasic muscles, which are responsible for quick movement, are examined for loss of strength.
- If a diagnosis of muscle shortening is made, in either one muscle or an entire muscle group, further palpatory examination of the muscle becomes necessary.

Paravertebral Palpation of the Skin

- The patient is positioned prone on the examination table. The examiner produces a skin bulge in front of the palpating fingers by gently pressing the index and middle finger against the skin. Applying a constant downward and cephalad force, the two fingers are pushed, along with the bulge in front, from inferior to superior on either side of the spine, along a line parallel and slightly lateral to the spine (Fig. **29**).
- Evaluate the ease of skin displacement or resiliency, moisture, and pain provocation.

Manual Diagnosis
Functional Examination

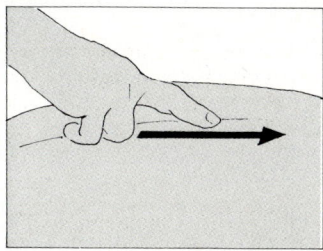

Fig. 29

- Findings consistent with and typical for a segmental or regional dysfunction include increased resistance to displacement, increased moisture production, and tenderness or pain of the skin.
- Erythematous changes can also indicate autonomic changes ("thick skin fold" test). In the skin-rolling test (Kibler fold), a skin fold extending just lateral to either side of the midline of the spine is formed between thumb and index finger of each hand (Figs. **30, 31**). Starting from below and following the course of the spine, this fold is rolled upward towards the patient's head. Again, the ease of displacement, skin thickness, and pain provocation, are evaluated.

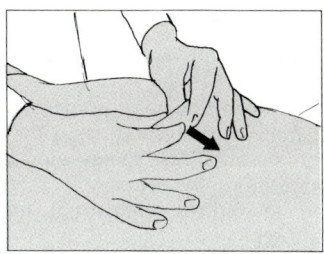

Fig. 30

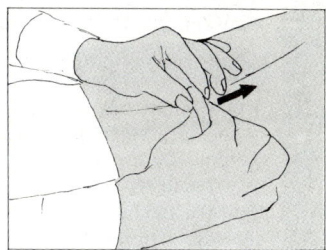

Fig. 31

Muscle palpation

- When examining the muscle by palpation, it should be done in its entirety, namely, from origin to insertion. The portion at the muscle–tendon junction is best palpated by following the direction of the muscle fibers (Fig. **32a**), whereas the muscle belly should be palpated in a direction perpendicular to the muscle fibers (Fig. **32b**).

Manual Diagnosis
Functional Examination

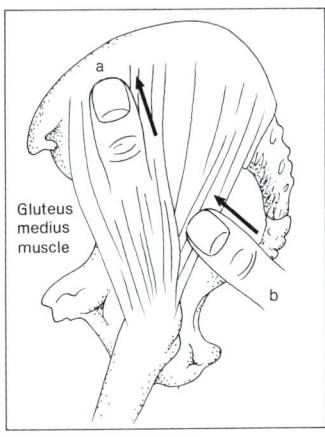

Fig. **32** Direction of palpation; a) at the insertion of the tendon; b) at the muscle belly

- Palpation of the muscle helps to distinguish between healthy, unaffected muscles and painful, pathologically tight muscle (taut, palpable band).
- Usually palpation is begun in the area indicated by the patient to be painful, be the pain present at rest or felt with movement or pressure.
- Once localized, the painful area should be described well, that is, in anatomic terms relating to certain landmarks.

Zone of Irritation

- The afferent source of the spondylogenic pain syndrome is primarily the intervertebral joint. Mediated through the central nervous system, changes in related soft tissue structures can develop reflexly as a result of permanently suprathreshold stimulations of the numerous mechanoreceptive and nociceptive receptors in the joint capsules and ligamentous structures.
- The first clinical manifestation is the zone of irritation.
- These zones of irritation are painful swellings, tender upon pressure, and detectable with palpation. Located in the musculofascial tissue in topographically well-defined sites, their average size varies from 0.5 to 1 cm. Its distinctive characteristic is that the appearance of the zone of irritation is directly related to the extent of a somatic dysfunction (functional disturbance) in a spinal segment, both temporally and qualitatively. As long as a disturbance continues to exist, zones of irritation can be clinically demonstrated, but should disappear immediately with the correction of the dysfunction. This fact is of great significance for the control of the therapeutic success.
- Let us emphasize that this is a term used to describe clinical findings established through the palpatory examination (Table **3**).

Manual Diagnosis
Functional Examination

Table 3 Important characteristics for the zone of irritation and spondylogenic myotendinosis in the context of the spondylogenic reflex syndrome

	Zone of irritation	Spondylogenic myotendinosis
Changes	Skin, subcutaneous tissues, tendons, muscles, joint capsule	Muscles, ligaments
Localization	In area of the disturbed spinal segment, topographically defined in region around spinous or articular processes	Muscles, ligaments (reffered pain?)
Time course (latency)	Immediate reaction to a segmental dysfunction	Apparent after a certain latent period
Qualitative palpatory findings	Decreased ease of skin displacement, increased tissue tension, localized pain	Increased resistance, less resiliency, tender upon pressure with radiation (trigger?)
Quantitative palpatory findings	Related to the degree of abnormal segmental function	Dependent on the duration of segmental dysfunction
Changes observed with successful treatment	Immediate decrease in quality and quantity	May disappear after a certain latency period (possibly reflexively)

Examination Techniques
Cervical Spine
C0–C1

Examination

Flexion and extension, passive motion testing.

Examination Procedure

- Patient sitting.
- The examiner fixates (stabilizes) the patient's axis with the index finger and thumb of one hand.
- With the other hand and arm, the examiner cradles the patient's head.
- Passive flexion (inclination) and extension (reclination) movements are performed (Figs. **33, 34,** respectively).

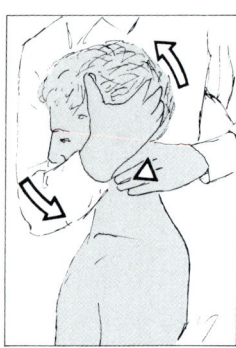

Fig. 33

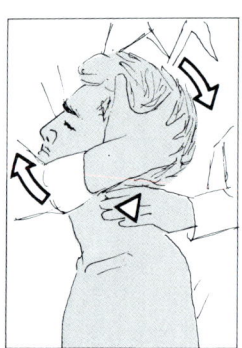

Fig. 34

Note

- The fixating fingers should not compress the soft tissues, especially not the muscles overlying the transverse processes.
- The range of motion is approximately 15–20°.

Pathologic Findings

- Decreased range of motion (motion restriction).
- Hard endfeel: indicates an articular degenerative cause.
- Soft endfeel: indicates the possibility of a shortening of the suboccipital muscles.
- Suboccipital pain during this movement may be due to segmental dysfunction (differential diagnostic considerations include instability at C0–C3, inflammatory changes).
- If autonomic symptoms or dizziness occur, a further neurologic work-up becomes necessary.
- Zones of irritation.

Examination Techniques
Cervical Spine
C0–C3

Examination

Axial rotation, passive motion testing.

Examination Procedure

- Patient sitting.
- The examiner introduces maximal flexion to the cervical spine.
- With the other hand placed broadly over the patient's mandible, the examiner introduces rotation to the upper cervical spine, alternating to either side (Figs. **35, 36**).

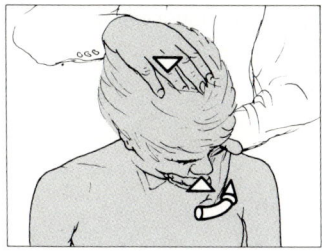 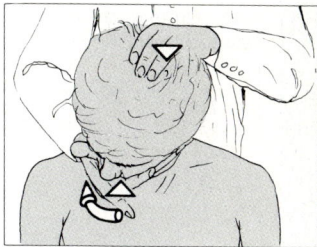

Fig. 35   Fig. 36

Note

- The physiologic range of motion for rotation to either side measures 40–45°.

Pathologic Findings

- Decreased rotation motion (rotation restriction).
- Hard endfeel: indicates articular degenerative changes.
- Soft endfeel: due to shortening of the suboccipital muscles.
- Suboccipital pain: indicates a segmental dysfunction.
- Vertigo at the extreme of the movement may occur, requiring further neurologic investigation (vertebral artery).
- Zones of irritation.
- In the presence of enhanced rotation: technically incorrect performance of this examination, or the patient may be recruiting additional movement. However, one should always consider the possibility of rotation instability in the upper cervical spine.

Examination Techniques
Cervical Spine
C1–C2

Examination

Axial rotation at C1–C2 (joint play), passive motion testing.

Examination Procedure

- Patient sitting.
- The examiner stands at the side of the patient and stabilizes the patient against his or her upper body.
- One hand gently fixates the patient's axis (C2) with thumb and index finger.
- The other hand cradles the patient's head such that the hypothenar and small finger make contact with the transverse process of the atlas (C1).
- The examiner introduces passive rotation movement of the head to its motion barrier (Fig. 37).

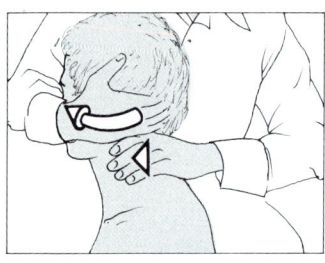

Fig. 37

Note

- Axis fixation must be maintained throughout the entire course of head rotation. Range of motion measures 30–45°.

Pathologic Findings

- Loss of angular mobility.
- Decreased joint play.
- Hard endfeel: may indicate articular degenerative changes.
- Soft endfeel: may be due to shortened postural suboccipital muscles.
- Pain induced with movement indicates a segmental dysfunction.
- The appearance of dizziness (possibility of instability, inflammatory processes affecting the cervical spinal joints, irritation of the vertebral artery).

Examination Techniques
Cervical Spine
C0–C3

Examination

Provocative testing (vertebral artery).

Examination Procedure

- Patient sitting.
- The examiner introduces a combination of cervical spine extension and rotation to one side.
- The patient is requested to look up at the operator's index finger placed in the direction opposite to that of rotation (Fig. **38**).
- It is observed whether there is appearance of nystagmus.

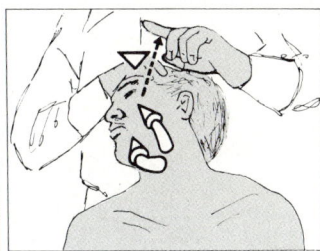

Fig. **38**

Note

- The patient should be maintained in this position for at least 20–30 seconds so as not to miss any latent nystagmus.
- This examination is performed to either side.
- If the patient complains of dizziness, nausea, or if there is unabating nystagmus, the examination should be terminated immediately.

Pathologic Findings

- Slowly progressive vertigo during the examination, occasionally accompanied by unabating nystagmus, primarily that of the crescendo type, may be due to a peripheral and/or central vestibular disturbance secondary to decreased blood flow in the vertebral artery distribution.
- Vertigo at the onset of the examination but improving during the examination, occasionally accompanied by nystagmus that resolves, may indicate cervical vertigo or cervical nystagmus. Further examination by the otoneurologist is indicated.

Examination Techniques
Cervical Spine—Cervicothoracic Junction
C3–T3

Examination

Rotation with extension, passive motion testing.

Examination Procedure

- Patient sitting.
- The examiner, standing behind the patient, stabilizes the patient's trunk against his or her thighs.
- The examiner places both hands flat over the patient's head in the parietal region.
- The examiner introduces passive cervical spine extension (Fig. **39**).
- In the second step, a passive, axial rotation to the head is introduced, alternating from one side to the other (Figs. **40, 41**).

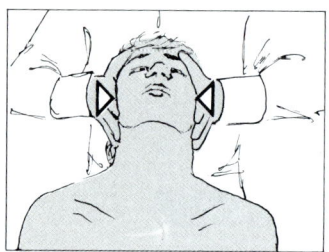

Fig. **39**   Fig. **40**

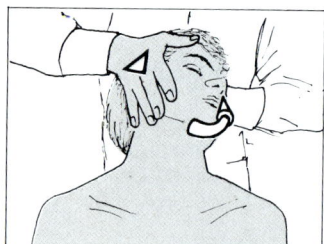

Fig. **41**

Examination Techniques
Cervical Spine—Cervicothoracic Junction
C3–T3

Note

- During maximal cervical spine extension, the upper cervical spinal joints become fixated (stabilized) due to increased tension in the alar ligaments.
- This allows selective rotation movement of the lower cervical spine.
- The symmetry of range of motion to either side is determined.
- Empirical measurements have been determined to be 60° of rotation.

Pathologic Findings

- Overall rotation restriction.
- Asymmetry in rotation of one side compared to the other.
- Rotation restriction with hard endfeel and pain at the barrier: indicates degenerative changes in the area of the midcervical spine (spondylosis, spondyloarthrosis, uncarthrosis).
- Soft endfeel: more likely due to shortening of the long neck extensor muscles or the longus colli muscle.
- Pain at the barrier (extreme of motion): probably due to segmental dysfunction.
- Vertigo with nystagmus: Suspect a decrease in blood flow or irritation of the vertebral artery (compare provocative testing of the vertebral artery, p. 33).

Examination Techniques

Cervical Spine—Cervicothoracic Junction
C0–T3

Examination

Flexion and extension, passive motion testing.

Examination Procedure

- Patient sitting.
- The examiner stands to the side of the patient and fixates the patient's trunk against his or her thighs.
- With one hand, the examiner fixates the head and introduces passive flexion to the cervical spine (Fig. 42).
- Now the hands are switched so that the upper hand can introduce passive extension to the cervical spine (Fig. 43).

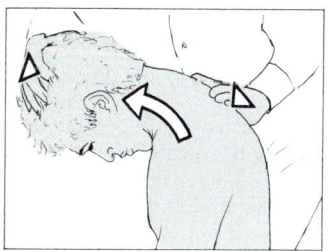
Fig. 42

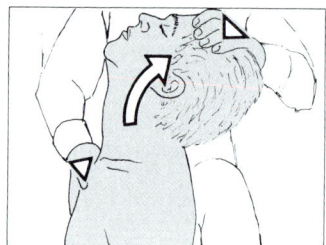
Fig. 43

Note

- Stop movement when the patient complains of spain (caution: instability).

Pathologic Findings

- Overall flexion restriction: indicates degenerative changes.
- Pain at the extreme (barrier) of movement.
- Soft endfeel: indicates shortening of the postural neck muscles.
- Localized, stabbing pain: may be due to segmental instability, especially with extension.

Examination Techniques
Cervical Spine—Cervicothoracic Junction
C0–T3

Examination

- Side-bending, passive motion testing.

Examination Procedure

- Patient sitting.
- The examiner stands behind the patient and fixates the patient's trunk against his or her thighs.
- One hand stabilizes the patient's shoulder.
- The other hand is placed over the parietal region of the patient's head.
- The examiner introduces passive side-bending in the direction opposite to that of the stabilized shoulder (Figs. **44, 45**).

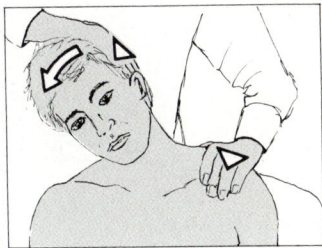

Fig. 44   Fig. 45

Note

- It is important to properly fixate the patient's shoulder (for evaluation of soft endfeel).

Pathologic Findings

- Overall side-bending motion restriction.
- Asymmetry of motion when comparing one side to the other side.
- Hard endfeel with degenerative changes.
- Soft endfeel: probably due to shortening of the postural neck muscles (trapezius muscle, descending portion; levator scapulae muscle).

Examination Techniques
Cervical Spine—Cervicothoracic Junction
C0–T3

Examination

Axial rotation, passive motion testing.

Examination Procedure

- Patient sitting.
- The examiner stands behind the patient and fixates the patient's trunk against his or her thighs.
- One hand is placed over the patient's shoulder for stabilization.
- The examining hand is placed in a viselike manner around the patient's head.
- Starting from neutral, the examiner introduces passive rotation to the cervical spine up to the motion barrier alternating between either side (Figs. **46, 47**).

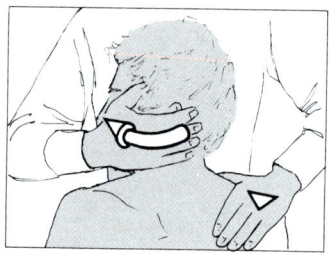
Fig. **46**

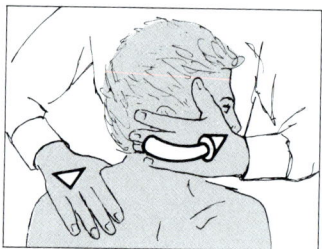
Fig. **47**

Note

- Normal rotation of the cervical spine measures 90° to either side.
- In this examination, it is important to compare the side-to-side movements, evaluating for asymmetry.

Pathologic Findings

- Overall rotation restriction.
- Pain at the extreme (barrier) of motion.
- Hard endfeel with pain: possibly due to degenerative changes of the intervertebral joints.
- Soft endfeel: may be due to shortening of the deep short cervical spine rotators and/or the postural neck and shoulder muscles (descending portion of trapezius muscle, sternocleidomastoid muscle, levator scapulae muscle).

Examination Techniques
Cervical Spine
C0–C3

Examination

Forced rotation of the axis.

Examination Procedure

- Patient sitting.
- The examiner fixates the patient's trunk laterally.
- The index and middle finger of the examiner's palpating hand are placed over the spinous processes of C2 and C3, respectively.
- With the opposite hand, the examiner fixates the patient's head over in the parietal region.
- The first step involves side-bending of the head to either side (Fig. 48).
- In the second step, axial rotation to each side is introduced (Fig. 49).

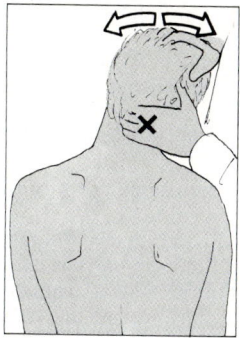
Fig. 48

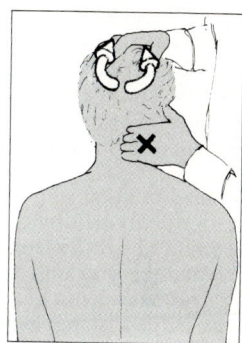
Fig. 49

Note

- With initiation of side-bending movement to one side, the axis immediately starts to rotate towards the same side (the spinous process moves in the opposite direction).
- In contrast, with axial rotation, the axis does not start to move until after the head has rotated 20–30°.
- Initial rotation takes place in the atlantoaxial joint.

Examination Techniques
Cervical Spine
C0–C3

Pathologic Findings

- Absence of forced rotation of the axis with side-bending movement may be due to a lesion of the ligamentous apparatus, in particular, the alar ligaments.
- Abnormal movements may be due to segmental instability in the upper cervical spinal joints.
- If the axis starts to rotate immediately with the initiation of axial rotation of the head, a segmental dysfunction at C1–C2 may be present (somatic dysfunction).

Examination

End (final) rotation of the atlas.

Examination Procedure

- Patient sitting.
- The patient's trunk is stabilized against the thigh of the examiner, who is standing behind the patient.
- The index finger of the examiner's palpating hand lies over the mastoid process, and the middle finger is placed over the transverse process of the atlas.
- With the opposite hand and arm, the examiner cradles the patient's head.
- Passive head rotation is introduced by the examiner up to the motion barrier (extreme of movement).
- In the second step, the examiner carefully introduces rotation to the head beyond the previously determined motion barrier.
- The springlike resiliency of movement of the atlas is evaluated (determining if the distance between the mastoid and the transverse process of the atlas decreases; Fig. 50).

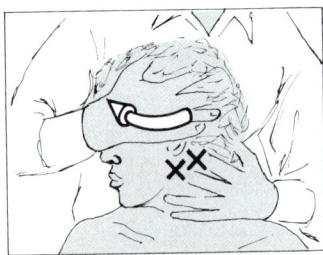

Fig. 50

Examination Techniques
Cervical Spine
C0–C3

Note

- Palpation of the transverse process of the atlas needs to be very gentle.
- Too forceful a palpation may provoke pain.
- The contact with the mastoid and the transverse process of the atlas must be maintained troughout rotation.
- The range of motion is rather small.

Pathologic Findings

- Absence of springlike movement at the atlas in endrotation: an indication of a segmental dysfunction (functional disturbance of the upper cervical spinal joints).
- Pain induced at the motion barrier along with a hard endfeel: indicates a segmental dysfunction (functional disturbance).
- Enhanced movement, that is, an increased distance between the transverse process of the atlas and the mastoid process, may indicate hypermobility (cervical spine injuries).
- Appearance of vertigo: may be due to irritation of the vertebral artery (see p. 33).

Examination Techniques
Cervical Spine—Cervicothoracic Junction
C3–T3

Examination

Flexion and extension, passive motion testing.

Examination Procedure

- Patient sitting.
- The examiner stands at the patient's side and fixates the patient's trunk with his or her thigh.
- With the fingers of one hand, the examiner palpates the patient's spinous processes of the lower cervical spine and the upper thoracic spine.
- The other hand is placed over the patient's head so that passive flexion–extension movement can be introduced (Fig. **51**).
- The goal of this evaluation is to determine overall mobility of the spinous processes and their movement in relation to each other.

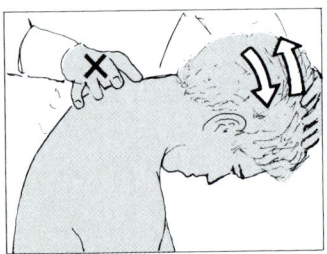

Fig. **51**

Note

- It is imperative to maintain good contact with the spinous processes throughout the examination.

Pathologic Findings

- Absence of movement of the spinous processes during this examination (that is, the spinous processes do not approximate with extension and/or do not move apart with forward flexion).
- Soft endfeel: often due to shortening of the postural neck muscles, including the descending portion of the trapezius muscle, the longissimus capitis and cervicis muscles, and the semispinalis capitis muscle.
- Hard endfeel may indicate degenerative changes at the intervertebral joints.

Examination Techniques
Cervical Spine—Cervicothoracic Junction
C3–T3

Examination

- Side-bending, passive motion testing.

Examination Procedure

- The examiner stands to the side of the sitting patient.
- The fingers of the examiner's palpating hand are placed segmentally over four neighboring spinous processes.
- The examiner places his other hand over the patient's head so as to introduce passive side-bending movement to either side (Fig. 52).
- Mobility and rotation of the vertebrae are evaluated.

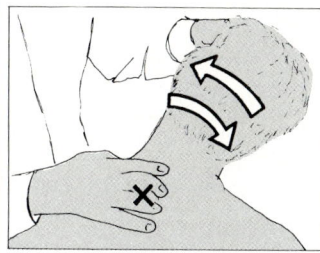

Fig. 52

Note

- The vertebrae rotate in the same direction as the side-bending.
- The spinous processes, however, move in the opposite direction.

Pathologic Findings

- Asymmetric range of motion during side-bending movement when comparing one side to the other.
- Hard endfeel: indicates articular degenerative changes.
- Soft endfeel: may be due to shortening of the postural neck and shoulder muscles (descending portion of the trapezius muscle, levator scapulae muscle).
- Absence of vertebral rotation (somatic dysfunction, spondyloarthrosis).
- Reversal of rotation: may be due to instability.

Examination Techniques
Cervical Spine—Cervicothoracic Junction
C3–T3

Examination

Axial rotation, passive motion testing.

Examination Procedure

- Patient sitting.
- The examiner stands at the side of the patient and fixates the patient's trunk against his or her thigh.
- The examiner localizes the spinous processes in question with the palpating fingers.
- With the other hand placed over the patient's head, rotation to either side is introduced (Fig. 53).
- Vertebral rotation is evaluated.

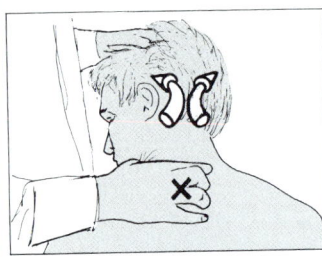

Fig. 53

Note

- Good contact with the spinous processes is to be maintained throughout the examination.
- Rotation of the head should be performed very slowly (caution: pain inhibition).

Pathologic Findings

- Asymmetry of rotational movement when comparing one side to the other.
- Hard endfeel: indicates articular degenerative changes (spondyloarthrosis) or segmental dysfunction (functional disturbance).
- Soft endfeel: often due to shortening of the deep, short cervical spine rotator muscles (rotator muscles, semispinalis muscles, multifidi muscles), and/or due to shortening of the superficial postural neck and shoulder muscles (trapezius muscle, sternocleidomastoid muscle, levator scapulae muscle).
- Absence of vertebral rotation: may be due to segmental dysfunction.
- Paradox vertebral rotation: may be an indication of segmental instability.

Examination Techniques
Cervical Spine
C3–C6

Examination

Axial rotation, passive motion testing.

Examination Procedure

- Patient sitting.
- Standing at the side of the patient, the examiner palpates the area over either facet joint of one spinal segment with thumb and index finger.
- The little finger of the other hand is placed over the neighboring superior articular process.
- Passive rotation is introduced by rotating the patient's head (Fig. 54).
- Segmental mobility in the facet joint is evaluated.

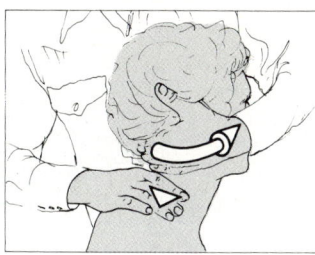

Fig. 54

Note

- It is imperative to assure good fixation of the inferior spinal segment.
- The soft tissues should be palpated carefully; too great a pressure should be avoided.

Pathologic Findings

- Asymmetric joint contours with individual movement.
- Absence of rotation movement in the superior segment: due to segmental dysfunction (degenerative changes, functional disturbance).
- Pain at the motion barrier: indicates a possible segmental zone of irritation.
- Soft endfeel: may be due to shortening of the deep rotator muscles (rotatores muscle, multifidus muscle, semispinalis muscle).

Examination Techniques
Thoracic Spine
T1–T12

Examination

Flexion and extension, passive motion testing.

Examination Procedure

- Patient sitting with arms crossed behind the neck.
- The examiner, standing to the side of the patient, reaches around the patient's trunk so as to stabilize it against his or her own chest.
- The fingers of the free hand, placed over the patient's thoracic spine, palpate the spinous processes.
- Passive flexion movement (Fig. **55**) and extension movement (Fig. **56**) are introduced.
- The examiner evaluates range of motion of the individual spinous processes.

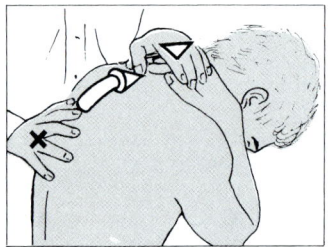

Fig. **55**

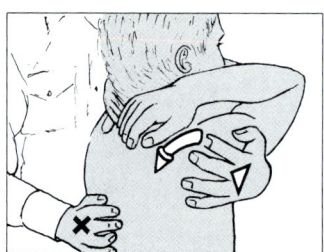

Fig. **56**

Note

- This examination requires accurate fixation and guidance of the patient's trunk.
- The examiner's fingers must maintain good contact with the spinous processes throughout the examination.

Pathologic Findings

- The spinous processes do not approximate (during extension) and/or do not migrate apart (with flexion).
- Pain at the motion barrier: may be due to segmental dysfunction.
- Soft endfeel: due to shortening of the postural back muscles (longissimus dorsi muscles).

Examination Techniques
Thoracic Spine
T1–T12

Examination

Side-bending, passive motion testing.

Examination Procedure

- Patient sitting with hands crossed behind the neck.
- The examiner, standing at the patient's side, fixates the patient's trunk against his or her own chest.
- With the other hand, the spinous processes are palpated (Fig. 57).
- The examiner introduces bending to one side by moving the patient's contralateral shoulder and trunk.
- Rotation of the vertebrae is evaluated.

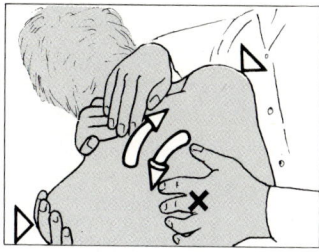

Fig. 57

Note

- It is imperative to maintain good fixation and accurate guidance of the patient's trunk.
- Good contact with the spinous processes must be maintained throughout.
- During side-bending, the upper thoracic vertebrae usually rotate in the direction of side-bending, whereas the lower thoracic vertebrae move in the opposite direction.

Pathologic Findings

- Absence of coupled rotation: may be due to segmental dysfunction (somatic dysfunction, degenerative changes).
- Pain at the motion barrier: may be due to a segmental dysfunction.
- Soft endfeel: due to shortening of the strong, deep rotator muscles (rotatores muscles, multifidus muscle, semispinalis muscle).
- Hard endfeel: due to dysfunction in the sternocostal joints.

Examination Techniques
Thoracic Spine
T3–L1

Examination

Axial rotation, passive motion testing.

Examination Procedure

- Patient sitting with hands crossed behind the neck.
- The examiner, standing to the patient's side, fixates the patient's trunk against his or her own chest.
- The palpating fingers make contact with the individual spinous processes to be examined.
- Rotation to either side is introduced by the examiner by moving the patient's contralateral shoulder and trunk (Fig. **58**).
- Mobility of the individual vertebrae is evaluated.

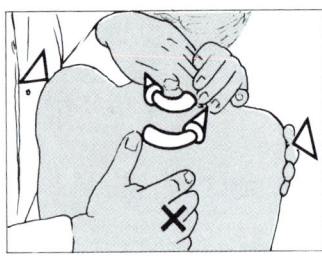

Fig. **58**

Note

- Good fixation and controlled guidance of the patient's trunk is imperative.
- Contact with the spinous processes must be maintained throughout the examination.

Pathologic Findings

- Absence of vertebral rotation (absence of coupled movements).
- Hard endfeel with pain at the motion barrier: indicates segmental dysfunction (somatic dysfunction, degenerative changes).
- Soft endfeel: may be due to shortening of the deep rotator muscles.

Examination Techniques
Rib I

Examination

Passive motion testing.

Examination Procedure

- Patient sitting.
- The operator stands behind the patient.
- The shoulder on the side to be examined is placed over the examiner's thigh.
- The examiner palpates the first rib with his or her index finger.
- The other hand introduces a combination of flexion and rotation of the cervical spine to the opposite side (away from the palpated first rib).
- This is followed by alternatingly side-bending the patient's neck from one side to the other (Fig. **59**).
- Mobility of the first rib is evaluated.

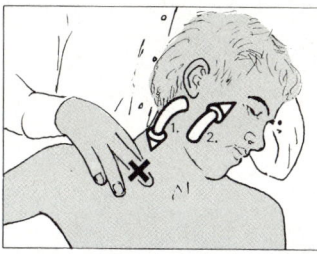

Fig. 59

Note

- Of utmost importance is a gentle palpation of the first rib (caution: brachial plexus).
- Compression of the soft tissues must be avoided (scalene muscles, nerves, and vascular structures).
- Too much palpatory pressure renders this examination valueless.

Pathologic Findings

- Absence of a spring-type movement of the first rib: may be the indication of a dysfunction, such as a somatic dysfunction in the first rib.
- Localized pain, occasionally referred to the shoulder and arm: may be indicative of scalenus anticus syndrome.

Examination Techniques
Ribs III to XII

Examination

Respiratory excursion of the individual ribs.

Examination Procedure

- Patient is prone.
- The examiner places both hands over the adjoining ribs.
- During inhalation and exhalation, individual rib mobility is evaluated (Fig. **60**).
- The same examination is then performed with the patient supine (Fig. **61**) or with the patient sitting (Fig. **62**).

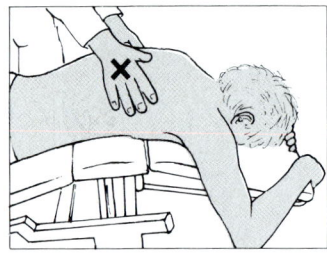

Fig. **60**   Fig. **61**

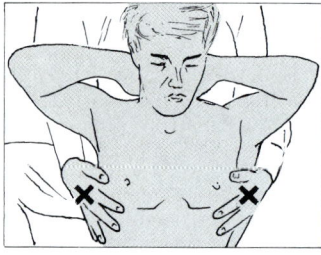

Fig. **62**

Note

- Good palpatory contact with the ribs is mandatory.

Pathologic Findings

- Asymmetric rib mobility: may be due to segmental dysfunction in the costotransverse joints.
- Pain more prominent in one position than another: also may be due to dysfunction in the costotransverse joint.

Examination Techniques
Lumbar Spine
L1–L5

Examination

Flexion and extension, passive motion testing.

Examination Procedure

- Patient sitting astride the examination table, with hands crossed behind the neck.
- The examiner stands to the patient's side and fixates the patient's trunk.
- The palpating fingers are placed over the spinous processes to be examined.
- Alternatingly, passive flexion (Fig. **63**) and extension (Fig. **64**) are introduced.
- Mobility of the individual spinous processes is evaluated.

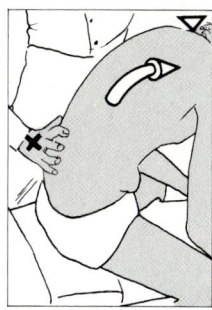
Fig. **63**

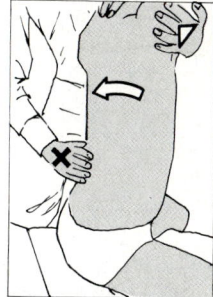
Fig. **64**

Note

- It is mandatory to maintain good bony contact with the spinous processes during this examination since the range of motion is rather small in the individual segments.

Pathologic Findings

- Generalized motion restriction, since the spinous processes do not undergo gliding movement.
- Soft endfeel: may be due to shortening of the postural lumbar muscles (longissimus dorsi, iliocostalis, and spinalis muscles).
- Pain at the barrier (extreme) of range of motion during flexion movement: may be due to a disk problem, that is, it may be a dysfunction localized to one segment.
- Localized pain during extension may be due to facet syndrome (spondyloarthrosis of the lumbar spine).

Examination Techniques
Lumbar Spine
L1–L5

Examination

Side-bending, passive motion testing.

Examination Procedure

- Patient sitting on the table's edge.
- The examiner, sitting astride the table next to the patient, fixates the patient's trunk against his or her own chest and holds the patient's opposite shoulder.
- The free hand palpates the individual spinous processes.
- Passive side-bending movement is introduced, alternating from one side to the other (Fig. 65).
- Vertebral motion of the lumbar spine is evaluated.

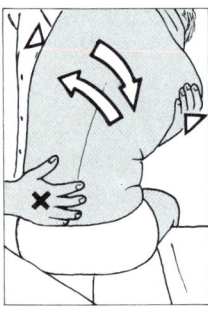

Fig. 65

Note

- The extent of side-bending in the individual segments measures approximately 6–8°.

Pathologic Findings

- Generalized restriction of side-bending movement.
- Localized pain at the motion barrier with hard endfeel: may be due to segmental dysfunction.
- Absence of coupled rotation or paradoxical rotation: may also be due to segmental dysfunction.
- Soft endfeel: indicates shortening of the postural lumbar muscles (longissimus dorsi, quadratus lumborum muscles).

Examination Techniques
Lumbar Spine
L1–L5

Examination

Axial rotation, passive motion testing.

Examination Procedure

- Patient in side-lying position, close to the table's edge.
- Both legs are flexed to 90° at the hip and knee joint.
- The examiner takes hold of the patient's leg just above the ankles (Fig. **66**). Both legs are lifted as far as possible.
- The palpating fingers are placed over the spinous processes of the vertebrae to be examined.
- By rotating the hip further, the mobility of the segments in the lumbar spine is evaluated (Fig. **67**)

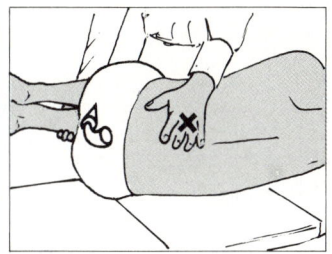

Fig. **66**

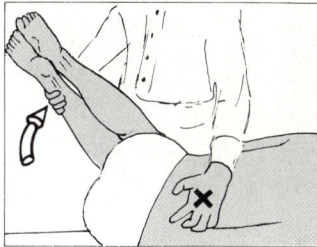

Fig. **67**

Note

- Correct execution of this technique is mandatory.
- Coupled rotation in the lumbar spine is rather minimal, measuring approximately 2° to either side.

Pathologic Findings

- Absence of rotation movement with hard endfeel: may be due to segmental dysfunction.
- Localized pain at the motion barrier: may be due to segmental dysfunction (spondyloarthrosis), as well as to hypomobility (osteochondrosis and/or disk problems).
- Soft endfeel: associated with a shortening of the deep lumbar spine rotator muscles (rotatores muscles, multifidus muscle, semispinalis muscle).

Examination Techniques
Lumbar Spine
L1–L5

Examination

Springing test.

Examination Procedure

- Patient is prone.
- The examiner palpates with index and middle fingers the joint processes of the lumbar vertebra in question.
- An anterior force is exerted (downward) against the spine through the hypothenar eminence of the other hand (Fig. **68**).
- The examiner and patient observe if pain is induced with this movement.

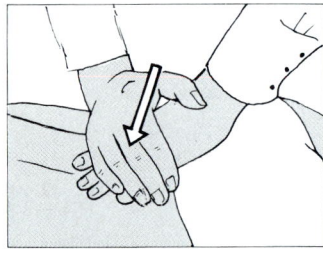

Fig. **68**

Note

- The reliance of this test is largely dependent on a clean palpatory technique of the articular processes.
- Palpation may be difficult due to the strong back muscles.

Pathologic Findings

- Localized pain induced with the anterior pressure: may indicate the possibility of segmental instability, diskitis, etc.
- Localized pain and/or referred pain: may also indicate diskopathy (osteochondrosis, especially in the L4–5, L5–S1 segments).
- Pain induced with superficial palpation: more indicative of a muscular insertion tendinosis.
- A positive test requires further differential diagnostic investigation.

Examination Techniques
Lower Lumbar Spine

Examination

Provocative testing of the iliolumbar ligament.

Examination Procedure

- Patient is prone.
- With the thumb, the examiner palpates the iliolumbar ligament between the posterior iliac spine and the spinous processes of L4 and L5 (Fig. **69**).

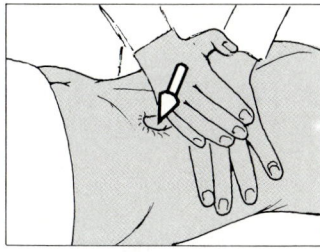

Fig. **69**

Note

- Palpation should be performed rather gently (painful insertion tendinosis at the transverse processes).

Pathologic Findings

- Localized pain with pressure: may be due to a functional disturbance in the iliolumbar ligament (segmental dysfunction, diskopathy).
- When pressing anteriorly (down) upon the spinous processes of L4–L5, the pain localized over the iliolumbar ligament actually becomes worse: may be due to spondylolisthesis.

Examination Techniques
Pelvic Girdle
Sacroiliac Joints

Examination

Sacroiliac joint nutation, spine test.

Examination Procedure

- Patient standing.
- The examiner, standing behind the patient, localizes and palpates the posterior superior iliac spine (PSIS) and the medial sacral crest at the same level (Fig. **70**).
- The patient is requested to lift the ipsilateral leg (hip and knee flexion).
- The PSIS moves inferiorly as a result of nutation (Fig. **71**).

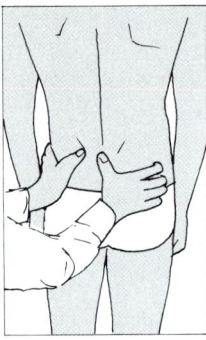
Fig. **70**

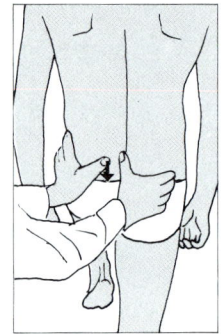
Fig. **71**

Note

- With unaltered sacroiliac joint movement, the PSIS usually moves inferiorly.
- In the presence of a sacroiliac joint dysfunction, the PSIS remains at the same level (i.e., does not move).
- Precise palpatory location of the PSIS is mandatory.
- The patient is allowed to place one hand on the back of a chair for support (balance).

Pathologic Findings

- Absence of sacroiliac joint nutation (PSIS remains stationary).

Examination Techniques
Pelvic Girdle
Sacroiliac Joints

Examination

Nutation in the sacroiliac joint (standing flexion test).

Examination Procedure

- The back of the standing patient faces the examiner.
- The examiner palpates the PSIS (posterior superior iliac spine) on either side with his thumbs (Fig. **72**).
- The patient is requested to bend forward slowly (Fig. **73**).
- Movement of the PSIS (movement of the ilia) is evaluated.

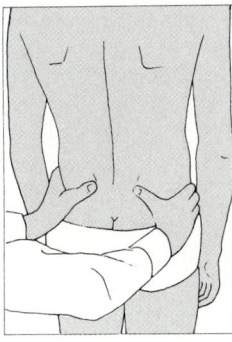
Fig. **72**

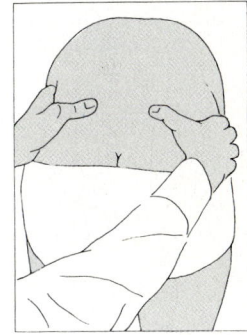
Fig. **73**

Note

- The ilium does not start to rotate until sacroiliac joint nutation (at the end of spinal flexion) has taken place. Physiologically, nutation should be symmetrical bilaterally.

Pathologic Findings

- Absence of nutation movement while the PSIS on the site of the somatic dysfunction actually moves more superior and anterior with forward flexion of the spine (*positive standing flexion test:* denotes the site at which the PSIS moves superiorly and anteriorly as compared to the other side).
- Differential diagnosis includes pelvic and hip-joint asymmetry.
- The differential diagnosis includes unilateral muscle tightening in the longissimus dorsi muscle.

Examination Techniques
Pelvic Girdle
Sacroiliac Joints

Examination

Sacroiliac joint, passive motion testing (joint play).

Examination Procedure

- Patient relaxed, in the prone position.
- The examiner palpates the sacroiliac joint and the short sacroiliac ligaments.
- The other hand is curved broadly around the ilium with the fingers placed anteriorly (anterior superior iliac spine region).
- Subsequently, the hand which is placed over the ilium introduces posterior movement to the ilium (Fig. **74**).
- The objective of this examination is the evaluation of relative movement between the ilium and sacrum.

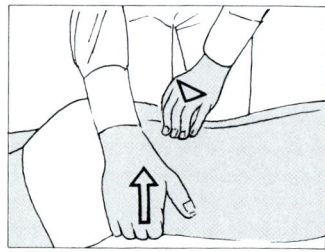

Fig. 74

Note

- Displacement of the ilium against the sacrum measures about 2–3 mm.
- Specific and well-localized palpation is mandatory.

Pathologic Findings

- Absence of sacroiliac joint displacement (hard endfeel): may indicate a functional disturbance in the sacroiliac joints.

Examination Techniques
Pelvic Girdle
Sacroiliac Joints

Examination

Patrick-Faber test.

Examination Procedure

- Patient is relaxed, in the supine position.
- The examiner standing to one side of the patient stabilizes the patient's pelvis on that side (fixation).
- The patient is then instructed to flex the opposite leg at the hip and knee joint, followed by external rotation and abduction in the hip joint as far as possible.
- The heel of the abducted leg is placed against the opposite knee.
- The distance between the patella and the table edge is measured (Fig. **75**).

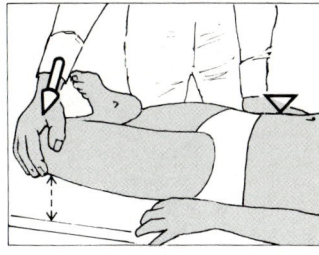

Fig. **75**

Note

- This is a rather nonspecific examination. In order to evaluate the sacroiliac joint, normal hip movement is a prerequisite.

Pathologic Findings

- Asymmetry in the distance between the patella and the table's edge when comparing both legs.
- In the presence of sacroiliac joint dysfunction, the distance between the patella and the table's edge is greater on the affected side than the noninvolved side.
- Hard endfeel: may be due to hip joint disorders (differential diagnostic exclusion of coxarthrosis must be made).
- Soft endfeel: may be due to shortening of the adductor muscles.

Examination Techniques
Shoulder Girdle

Examination

Sternoclavicular joint.

Examination Procedure

- Examiner stands behind the sitting patient.
- Starting laterally and inferiorly, the thumb of the palpating hand is placed at the inferior border of the middle third of the clavicle (Fig. **76a**).
- The opposite hand is then placed over the palpating hand so as to assist in introducing a translatory movement directed superiorly (Fig. **76b**)

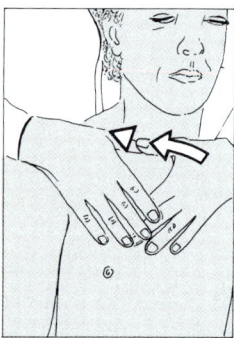
Fig. **76a**

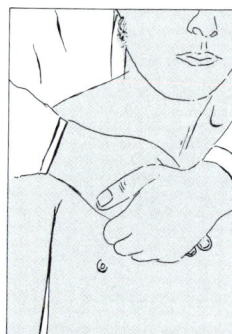
Fig. **76b**

Possible Pathologic Findings

- In the presence of functional disturbances as well as organic abnormalities in the sternoclavicular joint such as arthroses, the examiner perceives a hard endfeel.
- The patient may report localized pain.

Examination Techniques
Shoulder Girdle

Examination

Acromioclavicular joint, translatory motion testing.

Examination Procedure

- Examiner stands behind the sitting patient.
- One hand becomes the fixating hand, stabilizing the spine of the scapula as well as the head of the humerus and the coracoid process with the index and middle finger (Fig. **77**).

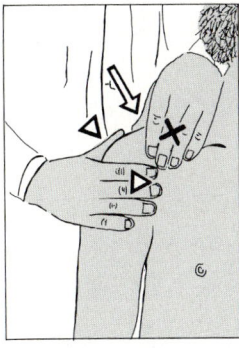

Fig. 77

- It is important to be very gentle when palpating the coracoid process, especially so as not to induce any pain.
- The other thumb palpates the lateral portion of the clavicle posteriorly and introduces translatory movement following the joint surfaces (10° in an inferior direction).
- In the unrestricted (freely mobile) acromioclavicular joint, translatory movement can be performed, ranging between 2−3 mm.

Possible Pathologic Findings

- Acromioclavicular arthrosis prevents translatory movement, and localized pain as well as pain radiating along the clavicle in the direction of the deltoid trigone may be elicited with this testing.

Shoulder Girdle

Examination

Axial traction in the glenohumeral joint.

Examination Procedure

- Examiner stands to the side of the sitting patient.
- One hand is placed broadly over the scapula to stabilize it.
- The opposite hand reaches the axilla from anteriorly such that the thumb overlies the major tubercle of the joint (Fig. **78**).

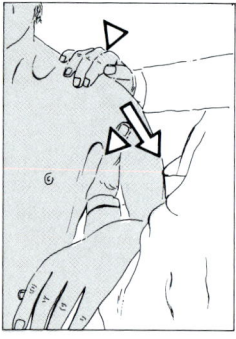

Fig. **78**

- Axial traction is introduced perpendicular to the joint surface.
- In the healthy adult, separation of the humeral head from the socket can be performed measuring about 3–4 mm.

Possible Pathologic Findings

- Shrinking of the capsule is usually accompanied by a hard-elastic endfeel.
- Decreased amount of traction.
- Patients with degenerative changes in the glenohumeral joint (arthrosis of the shoulder joint, omarthrosis) may actually report amelioration of pain with axial traction. This is a good indicator for mobilization treatment. In this situation, however, traction is also impeded.
- Increased traction movement with soft endfeel (instability, effusion = contraindication for manual therapy!).

Examination Techniques
Shoulder Girdle

Examination

Inferior gliding at the glenohumeral joint.

Examination Procedure

- Examiner stands next to the sitting patient.
- One hand gently reaches around the lower third of the patient's upper arm.
- With the elbow flexed 90°, the forearm rests on the examiner's forearm.
- The joint is abducted to 45° and forward flexed to 30°.
- With the hypothenar eminence placed over the head of the humerus, the examiner introduces inferior gliding movement (Fig. **79**).
- Physiologic gliding movement measures only a few millimeters.

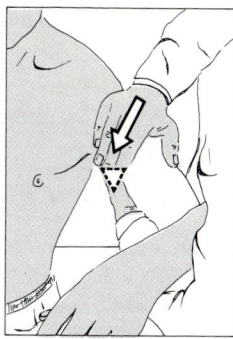

Fig. **79**

Possible Pathologic Findings

- In the presence of inferior joint-capsule shrinkage or injury to the glenoid labrum, the examiner will perceive an elastic endfeel. This is in contrast to arthrosis of the shoulder, where there is a hard endfeel, often accompanied by intra-articular crepitus. Pain may also be elicited, especially in the affected joint.
- Absence of pain despite shrinkage of the capsule.
- Soft endfeel in the presence of effusion.

Examination Techniques
Shoulder Girdle

Examination

Superior gliding in the glenohumeral joint.

Examination Procedure

- Examiner stands behind the sitting patient.
- The arm is slightly abducted and flexed slightly forward while the examiner places the hypothenar eminence over the head of the humerus of the patient.
- The other hand stabilizes the scapula posteriorly (Fig. **80a**).
- Starting from this position, the head of the humerus is translated superiorly in relationship to the scapula (in a direction parallel to the slightly concave joint surface).
- A similar translatory movement can be introduced through the hand placed in the axilla, keeping in mind that there is to be simultaneous axial traction as well (Fig. **80b**). With this technique, the translatory movement is primarily effected through the examiner's thumb.

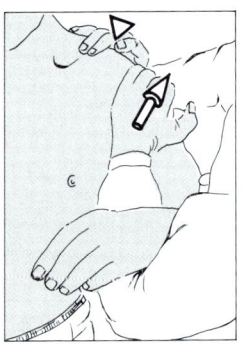
Fig. 80a

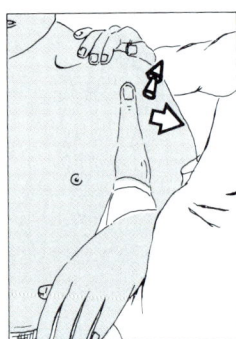
Fig. 80b

Possible Pathologic Findings

- Restricted translatory movements in the presence of shrinkage of the capsule, in particular, the posterior portions, as well as lesions of the glenoid labrum and arthrosis of the joint. The patient may report pain.
- Posterior instability allows increased translatory gliding movement. The endfeel is soft-elastic.
- In the case of a dislocated shoulder, posterior gliding is absent.
- Soft endfeel in the presence of effusion.

Examination Techniques
Shoulder Girdle

Examination

Anterior gliding movement in the glenohumeral joints.

Examination Procedure

- Examiner stands next to the sitting patient.
- The stabilizing hand is placed against the axilla from anterior. The tip of examiner's thumb may actually reach the lateral margin of the scapula.
- The remaining fingers stabilize the clavicle and coracoid process. The arm that is to be examined rests in a slightly abducted position on the examiner's forearm (Fig. **81**).
- The examiner introduces an anterior translatory movement by exerting a force through the hypothenar against the posterior portion of the head of the humerus.

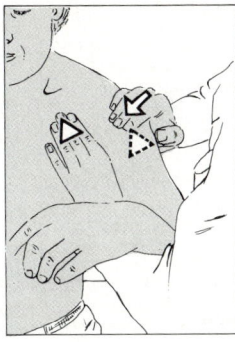

Fig. **81**

Possible Pathologic Findings

- If the anterior portion of the joint capsule has shrunk, a hard-elastic endfeel is noticed.
- Arthrosis of the shoulder may be associated with a hard endfeel. Painful crepitus may also be induced.
- Anterior instability, which is more frequent, allows abnormally large gliding movements, and the impression the examiner perceives is not unlike that of subluxation.
- Soft endfeel due to effusion.

Examination Techniques
Elbow

Examination

Motion testing of pronation and supination (forearm rotation).

Examination Procedure

- Examiner stands in front of the sitting patient whose hands are placed against the examiner's pelvis so as to be fixated there.
- With both index fingers, the examiner palpates the radial head as well as the radiohumeral joint.
- Starting from this position, the examiner introduces rotation movement simulating pronation (Fig. **82a**) and supination (Fig. **82b**).
- The palpating index finger follows the rotation movement of the slightly ellipsoid radial head, which becomes more prominent during pronation.

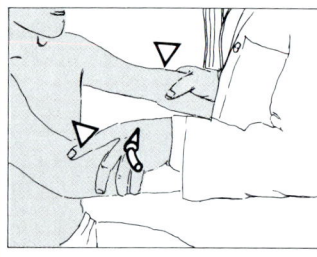

Fig. **82a**

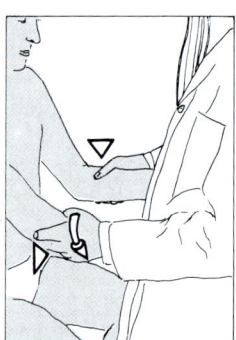

Fig. **82b**

Possible Pathologic Findings

- Functional disturbance affecting the proximal radioulnar joint causes movement to be asymmetric when comparing one side to the other.
- The joint space is either enlarged or diminished.
- Abnormally altered joint capsule (painful, more tense).
- Decreased range of motion.

Elbow

Examination

Radioulnar joints, translatory movement.

Examination Procedure

- The elbow of the sitting patient is slightly flexed.
- With thumb and fingers of one hand, the examiner stabilizes the ulna.
- With the other hand, the examiner palpates the radial head posteriorly with his or her thumb, and with the remaining fingers, palpates through the extensors (Fig. **83**).
- Starting from this position, anterior and posterior gliding movement is introduced.

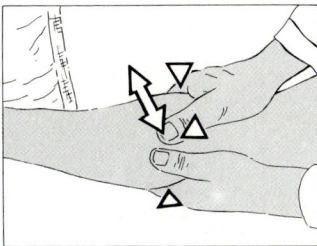

Fig. **83**

Possible Pathologic Findings

- Translatory movement is diminished in epicondylitis, especially when there are trauma-related degenerative changes. Pain may be elicited with the application of pressure.

Examination Techniques
Elbow

Examination

Traction and gliding movement in the radiohumeral joint.

Examination Procedure

- Examiner stands at the side of the table.
- The patient's arm is abducted to 40° in the shoulder (Fig. **84a**).
- The examiner stabilizes the arm proximal to the elbow joint (Fig. **84b**).
- The other hand, placed gently on the distal one-third of the forearm, introduces 30° of flexion at the elbow.
- Starting from this position, traction movement is introduced (Fig. **84b**).

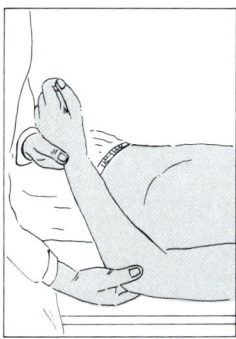
Fig. **84a**

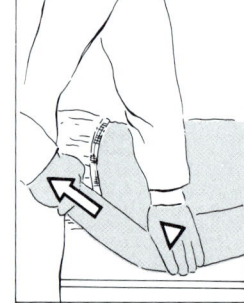
Fig. **84b**

Possible Pathologic Findings

- The examiner may perceive a hard endfeel, which is occasionally accompanied by pain, in particular when there are degenerative changes at the elbow joint.

Examination Techniques
Hand

Examination

Radiocarpal joint, translatory movement.

Examination Procedure

- One hand stabilizes the radius and ulna at the most distal portion (Fig. **85a**).
- The examining hand is placed such that it reaches around the proximal row of the carpal bones.
- The examiner evaluates traction movement. While introducing axial traction, translatory motion is introduced in a palmar and dorsal direction as well as in directions of the radius and ulna (Fig. 85b).

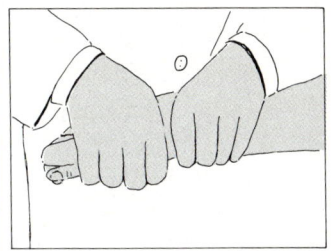

Fig. **85a**

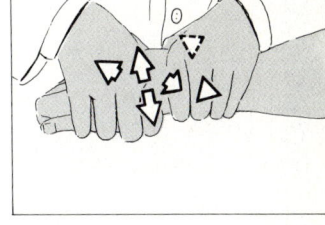

Fig. **85b**

Possible Pathologic Findings

- A functional disturbance affecting the individual joint causes a hard endfeel. Inflammatory changes may actually increase mobility which becomes a sign of instability. Pain may also be present.

Examination Techniques
Hand

Examination

Proximal carpal bones, palpation and angular movement.

Examination Procedure

- The index finger of the examining hand is placed over the radial fossa (the anatomical snuff-box).
- The index finger of the other hand is placed over the triquetrum along the ulnar side (Fig. **86a**).
- Introducing ulnar deviation of the hand (Fig. **86b**), the scaphoid bone moves towards the radius and becomes more prominent, whereas during radial deviation (Fig. **86c**), the triquetrum becomes more prominent as it moves closer towards the skin.
- Movement follows along the course of the concave joint surface of the distal radioulnar joint.

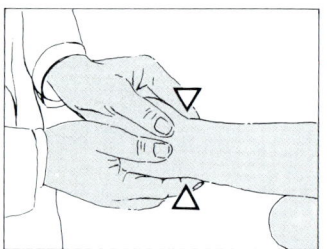
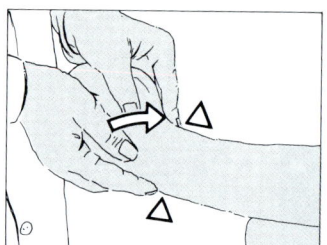
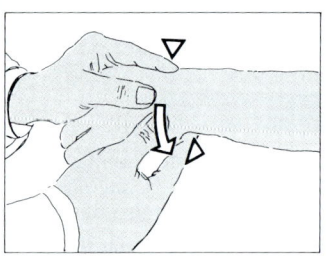

Fig. **86a–c**

Possible Pathologic Findings

- When there is a disturbance interfering with the radioulnar deviation movement, range of motion is actually decreased and the bony portions become less prominent on palpation.
- The scaphoid bone in particular may be subluxed especially with degenerative changes or inflammatory processes.

Examination Techniques
Hand

Examination

Palpatory and functional examination of the primary carpal bones (the scaphoid, lunate, triquetral, and pisiform bones).

Examination Procedure

- The patient's forearm is stabilized against the examiner's trunk.
- The thumb and index finger (Fig. **87a**) are placed over the scaphoid bone so as to introduce palmar and dorsal translation, with the radius kept stationary.
- Similarly, again with the radius stabilized, the lunate is moved in a palmar and dorsal direction (Fig. **87b**).

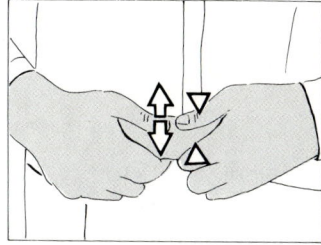

Fig. 87a

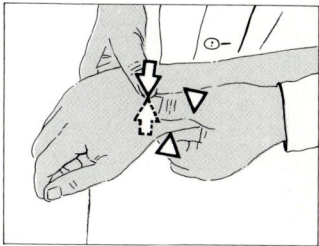

Fig. 87b

- On the other, ulnar side, the distal ulna is fixated while the triquetrum is moved in a palmar and dorsal direction.
- The pisiform bone is identified while the hand is slightly flexed (embedded in the tendon of the ulnar flexor muscle of the wrist). Movement in the radial and ulnar direction is introduced for evaluation.

Possible Pathologic Findings

- In the presence of a functional disturbance, movement is restricted and may be accompanied by pain.
- The scaphoid bone may be subluxed in the presence of degenerative or inflammatory processes.

Examination Techniques
Hand

Examination

Metacarpal joint translatory gliding movement, traction.

Examination Procedure

- The stabilizing hand fixates the scaphoid and trapezium bones with the index finger and thumb.
- With the fingers of the other hand, the examiner gently takes hold of the first metacarpal (Fig. **88**).

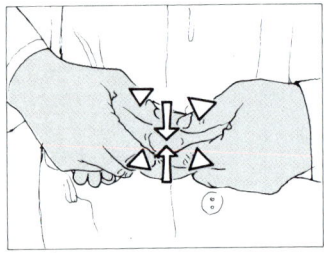

Fig. **88**

- In addition to traction, the bone is translatorily moved or translated in the palmar and dorsal as well as ulnar directions.
- Especially in situations of hypermobility, radial translation should be performed very carefully, as subluxation or even actual dislocation may occur.

Possible Pathologic Findings

- A functional disturbance may be identified when there is decreased or painful mobility. Instability causes increased range of motion, and radial subluxation may occur in arthrosis of the carpal bones.

Examination Techniques
Hand

Examination

Metacarpophalangeal joints, interphalangeal joints, translation testing.

Examination Procedure

- The forearm of the sitting patient is stabilized against the trunk of the examiner.
- The tumb and index finger of one hand stabilize the particular joint proximally.
- The fingers of the other hand are placed similarly over the corresponding phalanx, as close to the joint as possible.
- While introducing traction at the same time, the metacarpophalangeal joint is translated anteriorly, posteriorly, radially and ulnarly. Pure traction movement is also introduced (Fig. **89a, b**).

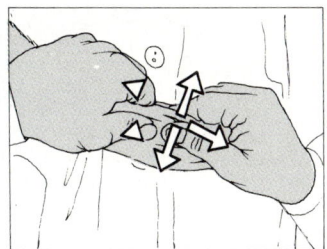
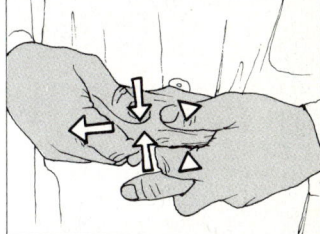

Fig. **89a**   Fig. **89b**

Possible Pathologic Findings

- Decreased gliding movement/traction after trauma or with degenerative changes (hard-elastic endfeel).
- Increased gliding/traction movement seen with effusion or instability, soft endfeel in the situation of inflammatory processes.
- Subluxation in an anterior/posterior direction is often posttraumatic and may also be seen with inflammatory processes.

Examination Techniques
Knee Joints

Examination

Femoropatellar gliding: superior–inferior, medial–lateral.

Examination Procedure

- With the patient supine, the hip and knee joints are somewhat flexed with a towel placed under the popliteal space.
- The examiner takes hold of the patella with his index finger and thumb and subsequently introduces movement of the patella in a superior and inferior direction (Fig. **90a**) and a medial and lateral direction (Fig. **90b**). This gliding movement should be performed with the muscles as relaxed as possible.

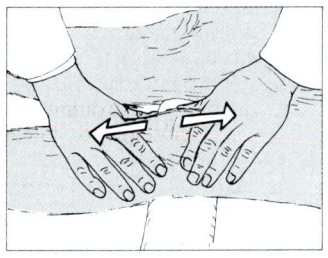
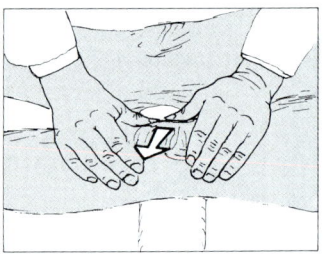
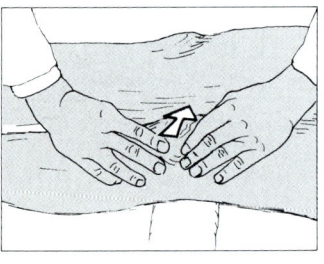

Fig. **90 a–c**

- It is emphasized that the femoropatellar joint should never be compressed when examining a patient who is suspected of having arthrosis.
- Range of motion is evaluated as well as endfeel, crepitus and/or grinding motion.

Possible Pathologic Findings

- Dislocation or subluxation.
- Crepitus.
- Decreased range of motion.
- Pain; Chondromalacia patellae.

Examination Techniques
Knee Joints

Examination

Examination of axial traction, anterior and posterior translation, axial rotation.

Examination Procedure

- Patient sitting at the edge of the examination table with the thigh supported but the leg distal to the knee hanging freely.
- With one hand placed over the malleoli, the distal leg is moved such that the knee is brought into its resting position (most loosely packed).
- While the examiner introduces axial traction, the thumb and index finger of the other hand palpate the medial and lateral joint space (Fig. **91a**). Of interest is the extent of traction possible (increasing the joint space).
- Starting from the same position, axial traction is supplied (Level 1, performed through the examiner's thighs). The examiner places both thumbs around the tibial plateau and subsequently introduces anterior and posterior translatory movement (**91b**).
- Introducing a medial and lateral pressure to the tibial plateau, axial rotation is evaluated (Fig. **91c**).

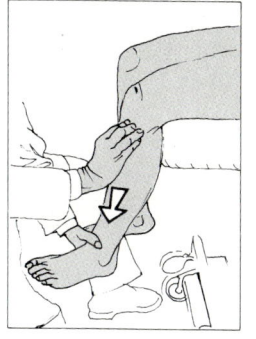

a

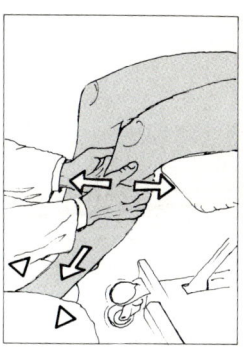

b

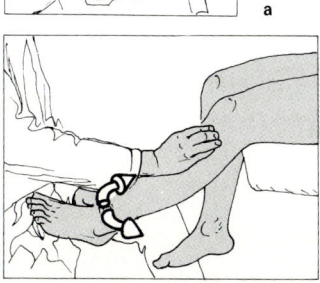

c

Fig. **91a–c**

Examination Techniques
Knee Joints

- When introducing gliding movement, not only the range of motion but also endfeel as well as the presence of pain are evaluated.

Possible Pathologic Findings

- Decreased traction/gliding movement with a hard-elastic endfeel.
- Pain.
- Crepitus.
- Increased gliding movement with soft endfeel (instability).
- Subluxation.

Examination Techniques
Knee Joints

Examination

Proximal tibiofibular joints.

Examination Procedure

- Patient is supine, and the leg is flexed to 60° at the hip and 70° at the knee joint. The foot is placed on the examination table.
- The tibia is stabilized medially with one hand while the thumb and flexed index finger of the other hand stabilize the head of the fibula laterally (Fig. **92**).
- Starting from this position, an anterior and posterior gliding movement is introduced.

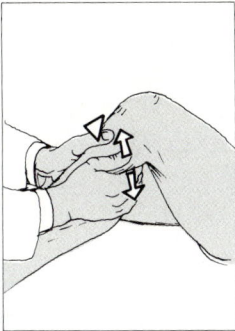

Fig. **92**

Possible Pathologic Findings

- The fibular head is displaced dorsally.
- Decreased anterior or posterior gliding with hard-elastic endfeel.
- Increased gliding movement with a soft endfeel.

Examination Techniques
Foot

Examination

Ankle joint (talocrural joint), translatory gliding movement.

Examination Procedure

- Patient is supine with the leg slightly flexed at the hip and knee joints.
- The patient's heel rests against the examination table. The examiner grasps the leg proximal to the ankle joint. The other hand stabilizes the foot (Fig. **93a**).
- A translatory movement is introduced to the ankle joint by moving the distal tibia posteriorly and anteriorly (Fig. **93b**).

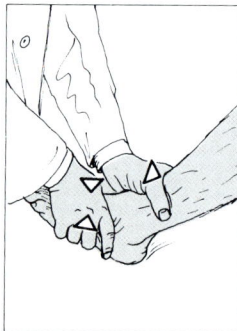
Fig. 93a

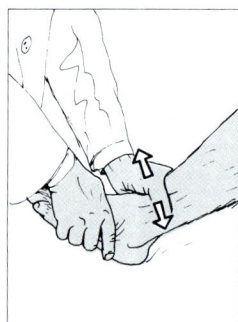
Fig. 93b

Possible Pathologic Findings

- Functional disturbances in the ankle joint may express themselves as decreased range of motion, hard endfeel, and pain.
- Decreased gliding seen with degenerative changes or after trauma; hard-elastic endfeel.
- Increased gliding movement with soft endfeel may be due to instability or inflammatory processes.

Examination Techniques
Foot

Examination

Tarsus, translatory movement in the talonavicular joint.

Examination Procedure

- Patient is supine, and the foot in a neutral position.
- The examiner stabilizes the talus dorsally with the thumb and anteriorly with the remaining fingers of the hand (talus with convex joint surfaces).
- The other hand grasps the navicular bone with the thumb placed at the dorsum of the foot and the other fingers placed on the sole.
- Under continued slight axial traction, the examiner introduces translatory movement both in the plantar and dorsal directions (Fig. **94**).

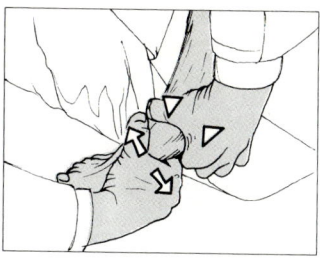

Fig. **94**

Possible Pathologic Findings

- Articular changes in the joint itself may decrease range of motion with hard endfeel and pain.
- Soft endfeel is noted with functional disturbances involving the talonavicular joint.

Examination Techniques
Foot

Examination

Tarsus, translatory movement between the talus and the cuneiform bones.

Examination Procedure

- The thumb and index finger of the examining hand takes hold of the navicular bone (stabilizing hand) (Fig. **95**).

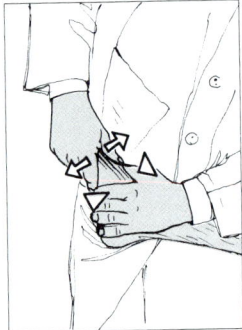

Fig. 95

- The thumb and index finger of the other hand take hold of the cuneiform bones I through III.
- Utilizing constant and simultaneous traction, the examining hand introduces movement, in a dorsal and plantar direction.

Possible Pathologic Findings

- A functional or organic disturbance involving the joint may cause a soft or hard endfeel, respectively. Pain may be provoked.

Examination Techniques
Foot

Examination

Tarsus, translatory movement, the calcaneal−cuboid joint.

Examination Procedure

- The examiner grasps the calcaneus inferiorly with the entire hand (fixation hand).
- With thumb and index finger, the examining hand is placed around the cuboid.
- Translatory movement in a plantar and dorsal direction is introduced (Fig. 96).

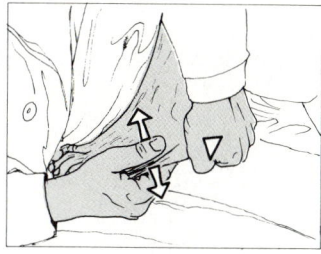

Fig. 96

Possible Pathologic Findings

- Functional or organic changes affecting the joint elicit soft or hard endfeel, respectively.
- Pain may be exacerbated with this movement in one or the other direction.

Examination Techniques
Foot

Examination

Tarsometatarsal joint, translatory motion testing.

Examination Procedure

- The cuboid is firmly grasped laterally between the thumb and index finger for stabilization.
- The examining hand grasps the 5th metatarsal firmly.
- Translation movement along with some traction is carried out in the dorsal and plantar direction (Fig. **97a, b**).

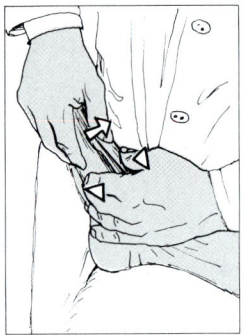 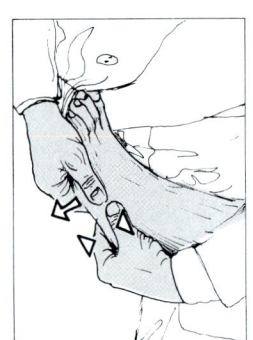

Fig. **97a + b**

- In similar fashion, the 4th metatarsal bone and other metatarsal bones can be examined: the first three metatarsal bones require stabilization at the cuneiform bones.
- For the first metatarsal joint, the hands are switched.

Possible Pathologic Findings

- Functional or organic abnormalities of the joint are accompanied by a soft or hard endfeel, respectively. Pain may be elicited.

Examination Techniques
Pectoralis major Muscle

Examination

Length testing.

Course

- In general, the pectoralis major muscle is divided into three parts, consisting of the clavicular, sternocostal, and abdominal portions.
- The line of origin extends from the anterior surface of the middle third of the clavicle, the sternal membrane, and the anterior layer of the rectus sheath in the uppermost area.
- The course is essentially horizontal with the abdominal portion being more vertical.
- Line of insertion is the intertubercular groove of the humerus and the greater tubercle.

Function

- Adduction of the arm and internal rotation.

Note

- This is a postural muscle with tendency to shorten.

Length Testing

- Patient is supine.
- The patient's thorax is stabilized by the examiner's hand placed broadly over it.
- Subsequently, the examiner introduces abduction and extension of the arm at the shoulder (Fig. 98). The extent of the range of motion and the tension in the pectoral muscle are evaluated.

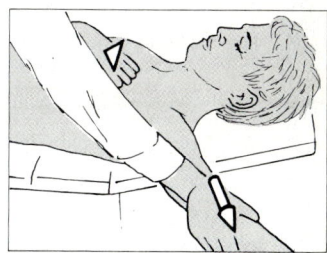

Fig. 98

Pathologic Findings

- Decreased abduction and/or extension with soft endfeel at the shoulder: probably due to shortening of the muscle.
- Pain during the arc of movement or at the extreme of movement requires further detailed examination to determine possible articular changes.

Examination Techniques
Trapezius Muscle

Examination

Palpation, length testing.

Course

- It is useful to divide this muscle anatomically and functionally into three portions: the descending, the horizontal, and the ascending.
- The origin of the trapezius muscle extends between the occipital bone and the spinous processes of C1 through T12.
- The line of insertion extends from the center of the posterior surface of the clavicle over the acromioclavicular joint to the superior border of the spine of the scapula. The fibers of the ascending portion insert at the inferior edge of the spine of the scapula.
- The muscle bundles arising from the occipital bone run sharply inferiorly, whereas the fibers of the central portion run almost horizontally in a transverse direction, and the fibers of the ascending portion run upwards.

Function

- Descending portion: elevation of the shoulder blade.
- Horizontal portion: adduction of the shoulder blade.
- Ascending portion: depression of the scapula.

Note

- The trapezius muscle is of great significance in the routine diagnostic work-up of functional disturbances.
- There is a close relationship between segmental dysfunctions affecting the thoracic and lumbar spine and individual muscle bundles of the trapezius muscle which have undergone myotendinotic changes (taut, palpable bands).
- Due to its subcutaneous location, the trapezius muscle can provide valuable information about texture, displaceability and possible myotendinotic changes (taut bands).
- Palpation of the muscle insertion follows along the direction of the muscle fibers.
- This postural muscle tends to weaken when involved.

Examination Techniques
Trapezius Muscle

Length Testing

- Patient sitting.
- The examiner stabilizes the patient's shoulder on the side to be examined.
- With the other hand, the examiner cradles the patient's temporal area.
- In the next step, and according to the course of the muscle fibers, the examiner introduces side-bending to the opposite side (Fig. **99a**) with rotation to the same side (1) or the opposite side (2) (Fig. **99b).**
- Evaluated are muscle tension, range of motion, endfeel, and the contour of the muscle.

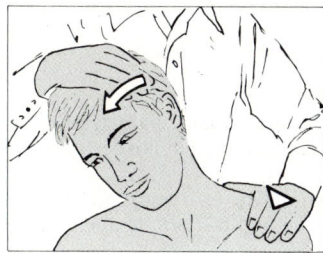
Fig. **99a**

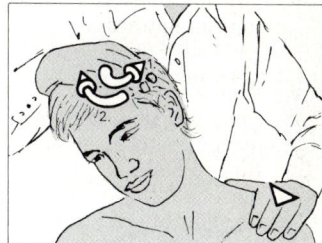
Fig. **99b**

Pathologic Findings

- Motion restriction with soft endfeel: indication of muscle shortening.
- Painful insertion tendinoses at the spine of the scapula or clavicle.
- Myotendinotic changes of individual muscle bundles ("taut bands").

Examination Techniques
Levator scapulae Muscle

Examination

Length testing.

Course

- Arises by four fasciculi from the transverse processes of C1–C4.
- Insertion is at the medial border of the scapula.
- The muscle fibers run laterally and inferiorly and, starting at C5–C6, are covered by the trapezius muscle.

Function

- Elevation of the shoulder blade.

Note

- This is a postural muscle which, when involved, tends to shorten.

Length Testing

- Patient sitting.
- The examiner, standing behind the patient, palpates the insertion of the levator scapulae muscle at the medial border of the scapula (Fig. **100a**).
- Starting from the neutral position, the examiner introduces a combination of cervical spine flexion and rotation to the opposite side (passive movement, Fig. **100b**).
- Evaluated are induction of pain, motion restriction, and tension in the levator scapulae muscle.

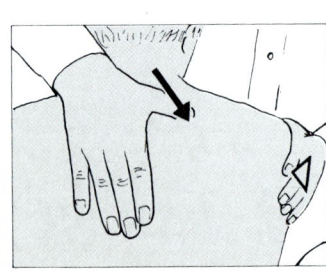

Fig. **100a**

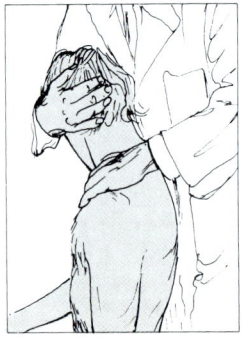

Fig. **100b**

Examination Techniques
Levator scapulae Muscle

Pathologic Findings

- Motion restriction with soft endfeel: may be due to shortening of the muscle.
- Quite frequently, there is localized pain at the medial border of the scapula.
- An insertion tendinosis which is painful, can often be palpated.
- If there is simultaneous myotendinosis affecting the levator scapulae and trapezius muscles (descending portion), there is localized pain at the intersection of these muscles (at T1 approximately three finger-breadths lateral to the spinous process).

Examination Techniques
Sternocleidomastoid Muscle

Examination

Length testing.

Course

- This large round muscle can be divided into the sternal and clavicular portions.
- The sternal portion originates at the anterior surface of the manubrium of the sternum.
- The clavicular portion originates at the superior surface of the middle third of the clavicle.
- This muscle courses in a screwlike manner obliquely across the side of the neck.
- The insertion extends from the mastoid process to the center of the superior nuchal line.

Function

- Bilateral contraction results in flexion of the head.
- Unilateral contraction results in side-bending towards the side of the contracted muscle and rotation of the head to the opposite side (typical presentation of torticollis).

Note

- This postural muscle tends to shorten when involved.

Length Testing

- Patient sitting.
- The patient's trunk rests against the thigh of the examiner, who stands behind the patient.
- The examiner palpates the clavicular and sternal origins of the sternocleidomastoid muscle with thumb and index finger.
- The other hand introduces maximal flexion to the head, maximal side bending to the opposite side with subsequent minimal rotation to the same side (Figs. **101, 102**).

Examination Techniques
Sternocleidomastoid Muscle

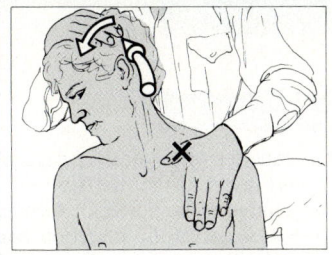

Fig. 101

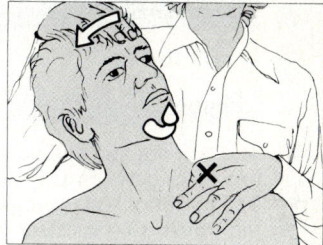

Fig. 102

Pathologic Findings

- Motion restriction with soft endfeel at the extreme (barrier) of movement with very prominent muscle contour: associated with shortening of the muscle.
- Slowly progressive vertigo: suspect circulatory compromise related to the vertebral artery.
- Vertigo occurring immediately with onset of the maneuver: may indicate the possibility of the cervical type of vertigo and requires further neurologic investigation.

Examination Techniques
Scalene Muscles
Anterior, Medial, Posterior Scalene Muscles

Examination

Length testing.

Course

- The anterior and middle scalene muscles originate at the transverse processes between C3 and C7 and insert at the first rib.
- The posterior scalene muscle originates at the posterior tubercles of the transverse processes of C6 and C7 with the insertion being at the anterior surface of the second rib. The fiber direction of all three muscles is lateral and inferior.

Function

- Bilateral contraction induces cervical spine flexion.
- Unilateral contraction results in side-bending of the head to the same side as the contracted muscle and also introduces cervical spine rotation in the opposite direction.

Note

- The insertions at the first rib are very tender when palpated.
- This is a postural muscle which tends to shorten when involved.

Length Testing

- Patient sitting.
- The examiner stands behind the patient and fixates the shoulder girdle.
- The index finger and thumb of one hand palpate the insertions of the scalene muscles along the first rib.
- The other hand introduces passive extension and rotation movement to the opposite side (Fig. 103) which introduces tension to the muscle.

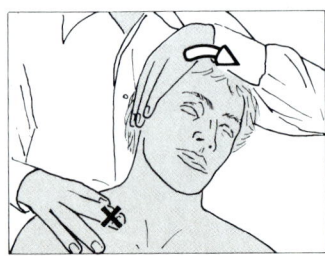

Fig. 103

Examination Techniques
Scalene Muscles
Anterior, Medial, Posterior Scalene Muscles

Pathologic Findings

- Soft endfeel at the motion barrier.
- Localized pain in the pectoral triangle, which occasionally radiates into the arm (the thoracic outlet syndrome should be included in the differential diagnosis).
- The "elevated first rib" is often seen with myotendinotic changes of the scalene muscles (hard, taut, palpable bands of the muscles).

Examination Techniques
Erector spinae Muscle, Longissimus lumborum Muscle

Examination

Length testing.

Course

- The anatomy of the longissimus and iliocostalis muscles, which form part of the sacrospinal system, is such that their origins at the pelvis cannot be differentiated from one another. Thus, just like a two-headed muscle, they share a common and remarkably broad origin.
- The longissimus lumborum muscle arises from the superior and anterior portions of the iliac tuberosity. It inserts via two tendons at each lumbar vertebra.
- The lateral row inserts at the posterior surface of the lumbar transverse processes.
- The medial row inserts at the mammilary processes.
- The longissimus lumborum muscle lies deep to the iliocostalis and longissimus thoracis muscles.

Function

- Bilateral contraction causes extension of the spine.
- Unilateral contraction results in side-bending of the spine to the same side as contraction.

Note

- The longissimus lumborum muscle is a strong muscle that can cause a functionally abnormal position (segmental dysfunction) in a lumbar vertebra.
- This muscle is a postural muscle, which tends to shorten when affected.

Examination Techniques
Erector spinae Muscle, Longissimus lumborum Muscle

Length Testing

- Patient sitting at the edge of the examination table.
- First, the muscle contours are evaluated for symmetry.
- The patient is then requested to bend forward.
- Both range of motion and endfeel are evaluated (Fig. **104**).

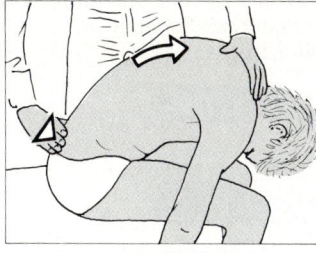

Fig. **104**

Pathologic Findings

- Prominent erector spinae muscle contours with readily apparent increased tension: an indication of muscle shortening.
- Significant loss of flexion motion in the lumbar spine with soft endfeel.
- Caution: Compensatory scoliosis may also be present in the case of acute disk herniation.

Examination Techniques
Piriform Muscle

Examination

Length testing, palpation.

Course

- Origin is at the anterior surface of the sacrum between the 2nd and 4th foramina.
- Starting at the lateral surface of the sacrum, the piriform muscle projects laterally through the greater sciatic foramen.
- Insertion at the tip of the greater trochanter.

Function

- External rotation of the thigh.

Note

- This is a postural muscle with tendency to shorten.

Length Testing

- Patient is supine.
- The hip on the side that is to be examined is flexed to 70°.
- Subsequently, the examiner introduces abduction of the thigh while maintaining pressure against the femur (fixation of the pelvis).
- The examiner evaluates whether there is motion restriction and pain provocation (Fig. **105**).

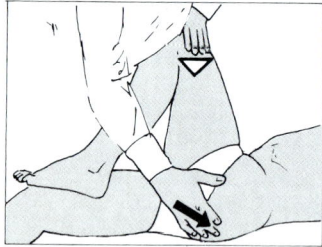

Fig. **105**

Examination Techniques
Piriform Muscle

Pathologic Findings

- Decreased adduction of the thigh with soft endfeel: may be an indication of muscle shortening.
- Decreased range of motion accompanied by stretch pain.
- During the length-testing procedure, the piriform muscle may also be palpated directly; when the muscle is shortened it has a hard, cordlike consistency.

Examination Techniques
Psoas major Muscle

Examination

Length testing.

Course

- The muscle originates at the anterior inferior surface of the transverse processes of L1 through L5.
- Portions of the muscle fibers may also arise from the lateral and anterior sections of the intervertebral discs of L1 through L5.
- Insertion is at the anterior half of the lesser trochanter of the femur.

Course

- Downward, alongside the lumbar spine (psoas shadow on X-rays), reaching the true pelvis, below the inguinal ligament with insertion at the minor trochanter.

Function

- Flexion of the thigh, and some participation in adduction and external rotation of the thigh.
- Unilateral contraction causes both the pelvis and trunk to rotate in the opposite direction.

Note

- This is a postural muscle which tends to shorten when affected.

Length Testing

- Patient is prone.
- The examiner stabilizes the patient's pelvis by pressing one hand flat against the pelvis in the direction of the examination table.
- The other hand grasps the patient's thigh.
- Extension is introduced to the ipsilateral hip joint by moving the thigh upward (Fig. 106).
- The examiner observes the behavior at the thoracolumbar junction.

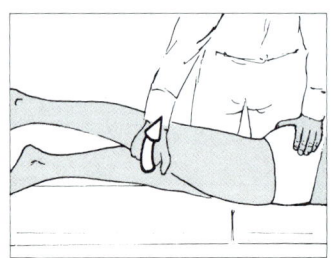

Fig. 106

Examination Techniques
Psoas major Muscle

Pathologic Findings

- Restricted hip extension with soft endfeel: most likely due to shortening of the psoas major muscle.
- Restricted hip extension with hard endfeel: may be due to degenerative changes within the joint itself. Sacroiliac joint function must be excluded.
- Prominent retraction of the thoracolumbar area; indicates significant shortening of the psoas major muscle.

Variation

- Patient standing.
- The height of the examination table is adjusted exactly to the height of the standing patient's ischium.
- The patient actively flexes the hip and knee.
- Guided by the examiner, the patient then reclines onto the examination table.
- One knee is brought up towards the chest so as to reverse the lumbar lordosis (fixation in this position).
- The leg that is being examined hangs freely off the table (Fig. **107**).

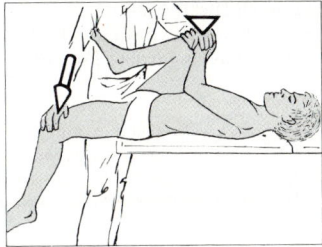

Fig. **107**

Pathologic Findings

- During the positioning phase, the free leg actually rises above the horizontal plane of the table.
- Soft endfeel when pressing the free leg downward.
- If the rectus femoris muscle is shortened at the same time, the knee will extend as well.

Examination Techniques
Rectus femoris Muscle

Examination

Length testing.

Course

- Origin is at the anterior inferior iliac spine and the upper rim of the acetabulum of the hip joint. Insertion is at the patella within its retinaculum.

Function

- The rectus femoris muscle is part of the quadriceps femoris system.
- Knee extension.

Note

- This is a postural muscle which tends to shorten when affected.

Length Testing

- Patient is prone.
- The patient's pelvis is fixated by one of the examiner's hands pushing against the sacrum in direction of the table.
- With the other hand, the examiner flexes the patient's knee, evaluating simultaneous movement at the pelvis girdle (Fig. **108**).

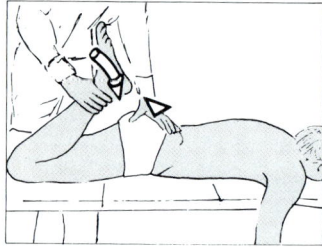

Fig. 108

Examination Techniques
Rectus femoris Muscle

Pathologic Findings

- With progressive knee flexion, the patient's pelvis on the tested side begins to lift off the examination table as a result of hip flexion due to a shortened rectus femoris muscle.
- In a differential diagnosis, this must be distinguished from nerve root irritation (upper lumbar spine — reversed Lasègue sign).

Note

- The length of the rectus femoris muscle can be tested at the same time as when examining the hip flexor muscles (see p. 97 and Fig. **109**).
- If there is shortening of the rectus femoris muscle, forced knee flexion causes the thigh to continue to rise above the horizontal line.

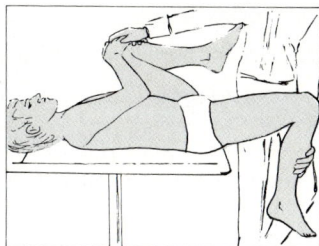

Fig. **109**

Examination Techniques
Hamstring Muscles
Biceps femoris, Semitendinosus Muscle, Semimembranosus Muscle

Examination

Length testing.

Course

- All three muscles arise from the ischial tuberosity. The short head of the biceps femoris has an additional attachment at the posterior surface of the mid-femur. The biceps femoris inserts at the head of the fibula.
- The semitendinosus and semimembranosus muscles insert at the pes anserinus and the lateral joint capsule of the knee.

Function

- Flexion of the leg at the knee and external rotation of the leg when the knee is flexed.

Note

- This is a postural muscle which tends to shorten when affected.

Length Testing

- Patient is supine.
- The examiner places both hands over the leg proximal to the patella and introduces passive hip flexion (Fig. **110**).
- There should be no knee flexion whatsoever.
- It may be helpful to fixate the patient's pelvis with a belt.

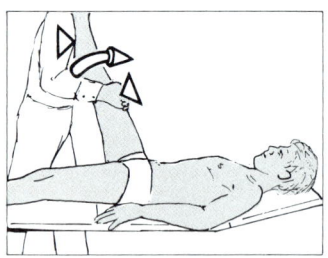

Fig. **110**

Examination Techniques
Hamstring Muscles
Biceps femoris, Semitendinosus Muscle
Semimembranosus Muscle

Pathologic Findings

- Loss of flexion motion at the hip with the knee extended and a soft endfeel: clear indication of shortening of the hamstring muscles ("pseudo-Lasègue sign").
- Loss of hip flexion with the knee extended and hard endfeel: may indicate a possible root irritation in the lumbar spine with root irritation secondary to a herniated disk.
- Degenerative changes affecting the hip must be excluded.
- Decreased hip flexion with a hard endfeel along with pain in the lumbar spine: most likely due to root irritation secondary to a ruptured lumbar disk.

Examination Techniques
Abdominal Muscles
Transversus abdominis Muscle,
Rectus abdominis Muscle,
External and Internal Oblique Muscles

Examination

Strength and endurance testing.

Course

- Due to their anatomic arrangement, the superficial abdominal muscles function very effectively as a unit.

Function

- With the pelvis fixed, both oblique abdominal muscles produce forward flexion to the spine. Unilateral oblique muscle contraction causes the thorax to be rotated into the direction opposite to that of muscle contraction. It is also involved when performing Valsalva maneuver.
- The rectus abdominus muscle causes the spine to flex and plays a major role in the Valsalva maneuver.

Note

- These are phasic muscles which have a tendency to weaken when affected.

Strength Testing

- Patient is supine, with the legs slightly flexed at hip and knees (to eliminate psoas major muscle action).
- The arms are then elevated slightly (Fig. **111**).
- The patient is requested to lift both the head and upper thoracic spine (down to the shoulder blades) off the examination table (Fig. **112**).
- The patient is requested to remain in this position for 30 seconds.

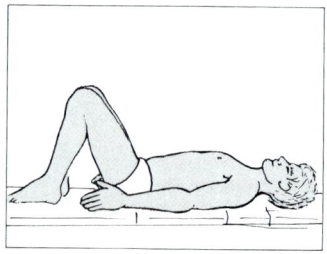

Fig. **111**   Fig. **112**

Examination Techniques
Abdominal Muscles
Transversus abdominis Muscle,
Rectus abdominis Muscle,
External and Internal Oblique Muscles

Pathologic Findings

- The patient is unable to assume the requested position.
- If the patient is able to assume the requested position, he or she is unable to maintain it for 30 seconds.
- The patient is unable to maintain his or her feet on the examination table during this test.

Examination Techniques
Gluteus maximus Muscle

Examination

Strength testing.

Course

- The gluteus maximus muscle can be divided into a superficial and deep layer.
- The line of origin for this muscle extends from the iliac crest via the posterior superior iliac spine to the lateral sacral line to the coccyx.
- The course of the muscle is in a lateral and inferior direction.
- The superior portions pass into the iliotibial band at the level of the greater trochanter whereas the inferior fibers insert at the gluteal tuberosity of the femur (thus forming a line of insertion that is 10 cm long).

Function

- Extension of the hip.
- Abduction and external rotation of the thigh.

Note

- This is a phasic muscle which tends to weaken when affected.

Strength Testing

- Patient is prone; the knee is extended to 90° (so as to eliminate hamstring function).
- The patient is then requested to lift the thigh off the table, at least 10–15 cm (Fig. **113**).
- The patient should be able to maintain this position for at least 8–10 seconds.

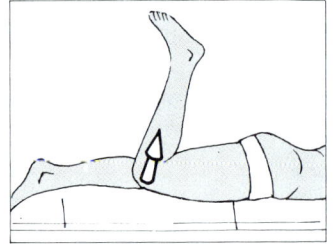

Fig. **113**

Pathologic Findings

- The patient is unable to assume the starting position for this examination.
- The patient is able to assume the position but unable to maintain it for 8–10 seconds.

Examination Techniques
Gluteus medius Muscle

Examination

Strength testing.

Course

- Origin is at the triangle formed by the anterior and posterior gluteal lines and the external lip of the iliac crest.
- This muscle is fan-shaped, and the overall course is lateral and inferior.
- The insertion is at the outer surface of the greater trochanter.

Function

- Abduction of the thigh.
- The deeper fibers cause flexion and internal rotation of the thigh.
- The superficial fibers are involved in extension and external rotation of the thigh.

Note

- This is a phasic muscle which tends to weaken when affected.

Strength Testing

- Patient in side-lying position.
- The knee is flexed to 90° (to eliminate action of the tensor fasciae latae muscle).
- In the second step, the patient is requested to abduct the hip (to 30–45°).
- Maintain this position for 8–10 seconds (Fig. **114**).

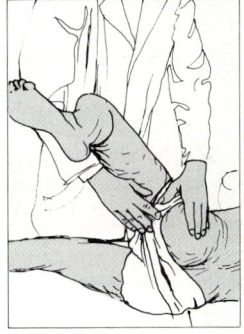

Fig. **114**

Pathologic Findings

- Patient is unable to perform the maneuver at all.
- The patient returns to neutral position before the 8–10 seconds have elapsed.
- Compensatory movement of the abducted leg by substituting with hip flexion.

Examination Techniques
Cervical Spine
Zones of Irritation C0, C1

Localization

- The zones of irritation of C0 and C1 are situated in the occipital region, related to the occiput and atlas.
- C0 is lateral and superior to the superior end of the mastoid notch whereas C1 is medial and inferior to it (Fig. **115**).

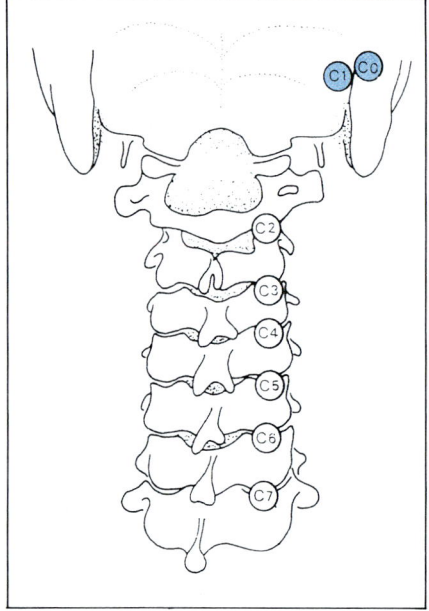

Fig. **115** Zones of irritation in the cervical spine region

Palpation

- The palpating finger localizes the bare bony part (no muscle attachments) located between the splenius capitis and obliques capitis superior muscles.

Note

- As it is difficult to differentiate these zones of irritation from insertion tendinoses of the numerous muscles originating at this location, provocative testing may need to be done.

Examination Techniques
Cervical Spine
Zones of Irritation C2–C7

Localization

- The individual zones of irritation are located over their respective intervertebral joints (Fig. **116**).

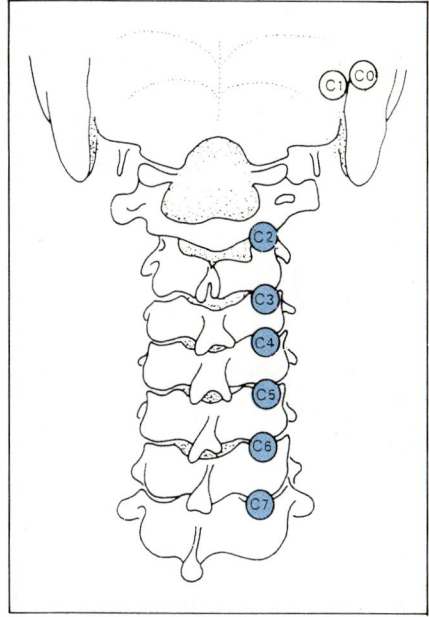

Fig. **116** Zones of irritation in the cervical spine region

Palpation

- The palpating fingers make contact with the spinous processes.
- In the next step, the fingers glide laterally over the strong semispinalis capitis muscle (approximately 2 cm).
- A groove formed by the semispinalis capitis and longissimus capitis muscles allows the palpating fingers to go deeper so as to palpate the intervertebral joints.

Note

- Localization of the individual zone of irritation is such that it is found one finger-breadth superior to the respective spinous process (i.e., irritation zone of C2 is one finger-breadth superior to the inferior edge of the spinous process of C2).

Examination Techniques
Cervical Spine
Zones of Irritation C2–C7

Provocative Testing

- In general, all zones of irritation in the cervical spine respond to provocative testing.
- A decrease of pain perception or any palpable tissue response indicates the appropriate therapeutic direction for the segment in question (Fig. **117**).

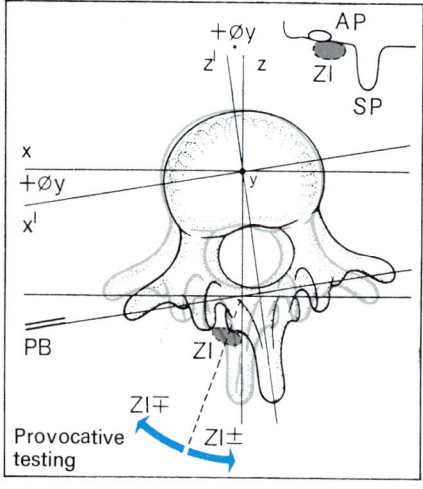

Fig. **117** Provocative tests: quantitative changes at the zone of irritation.
ZI zone of irritation
SP spinus process
AP articular pillar
PB pathologic motion barrier
$z-z' = +\emptyset y$
$x-x' = +\emptyset y$

Examination Techniques
Cervical Spine
Zones of Irritation C2–C7

Procedure

- The palpating finger remains in contact throughout the examination without exerting too much pressure.
- The examiner introduces passive rotation to the cervical spine to either side (Figs. **118, 119**).
- Both quantitative (patient response to pain) and qualitative (examiner response) changes of the zones of irritation are taken into account.
- These principles also apply to all other zones of irritation in the spine.

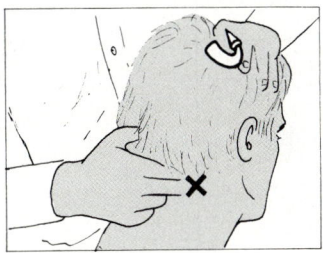

Fig. **118**

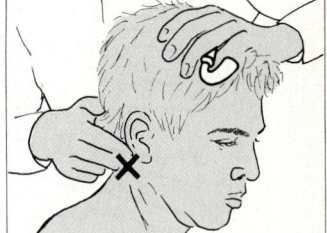

Fig. **119**

Examination Techniques
Thoracic Spine
Zones of Irritation T1–T12

Localization

- Localized at the transverse process of the thoracic vertebra at the level of the costotransverse joint (Fig. **120**).

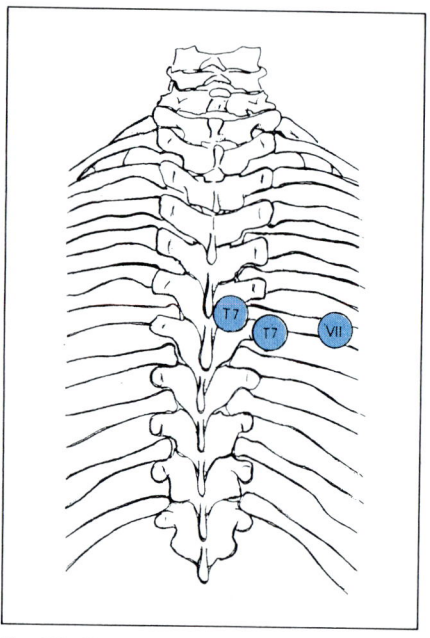

Fig. **120** Zones of irritation in the region of the thorax and ribs (example: T 7)

Examination Techniques
Thoracic Spine
Zones of Irritation T1–T12

Palpation

- Patient is relaxed, in the prone position.
- Patient is positioned such that thoracic kyphosis becomes somewhat exaggerated.
- Starting laterally, the palpating thumbs move medially along the course of one rib on either side, thereby displacing the longissimus system medially (Fig. **121**).

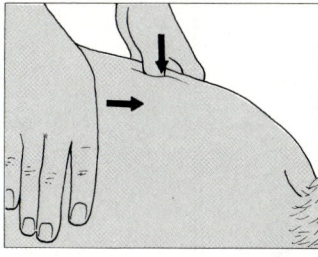

Fig. **121**

Note

- In the midthoracic spine, the transverse process is located three finger-breadths superior to that of its respective spinous process.
- In the upper and lower portions of the thoracic spine, the difference between the level of the transverse process and the spinous process is two finger-breadths.

Examination Techniques
Thoracic Spine
Zones of Irritation at the Ribs

Localization

- In the region of the costal angle, between the longissimus muscle and the iliocostalis thoracis muscle (Fig. **122**).

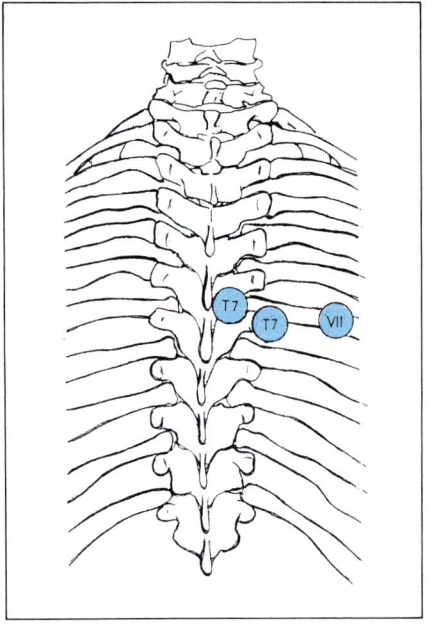

Fig. **122** Zones of irritation in the region of the thorax and ribs (example: I 7)

Palpation

- Patient is prone.
- The thoracic kyphosis is somewhat exaggerated through appropriate positioning.
- The palpating thumb localizes the angle of the rib by moving two finger-breadths laterally from the transverse process of the respective vertebral.
- Palpation is in a posterior–inferior direction.

Examination Techniques
Lumbar Spine
Zones of Irritation L1–L5

Localization

- Transverse processes of the respective lumbar vertebrae (costal processes; Fig. **123**).

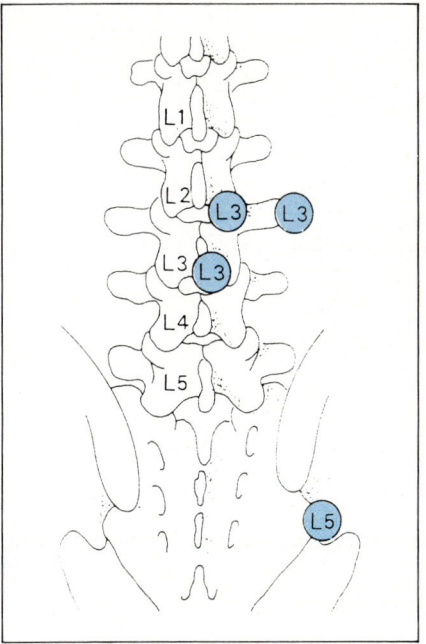

Fig. **123** Zones of irritation in the lumbar spine region (example L3)

Examination Techniques
Lumbar Spine
Zones of Irritation L1–L5

Palpation

- Patient is prone.
- The palpating thumb localizes the specific transverse process of the lumbar vertebra in question (make good bony contact).
- Starting laterally, the examiner moves medially between the iliocostalis lumborum muscle and the oblique abdominal muscles (Fig. **124**).

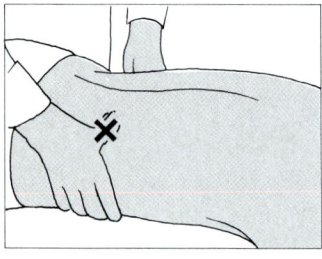

Fig. **124**

Note

- The transverse process is located approximately two fingerbreadths superior to its respective spinous process.
- Palpation of the transverse processes of L5 is more difficult.
- Zones of irritation must be differentiated from insertion tendinoses of the lumbar musculature.

Examination Techniques
Sacroiliac Joint and Pelvis
Zones of Irritation S1–S3

Localization

- In the area of the lateral portion of the sacral crest, located along an imaginary line connecting the posterior superior iliac spine (PSIS) and the sacral horn (Fig. **125**).
- S1 is localized approximately 1 cm below the tip of the PSIS.
- S3 is approximately at the level of the sacral horn.
- S2 is in between S1 and S3.

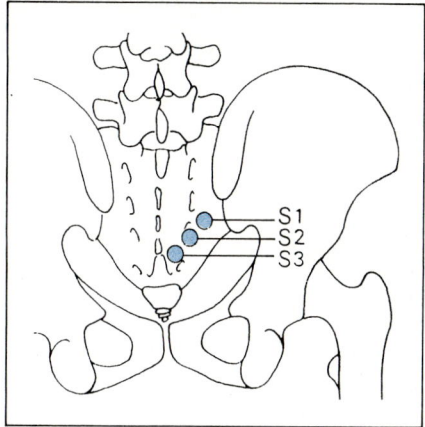

Fig. **125** Zones of irritation at the sacrum

Palpation

- Patient is relaxed, in the prone position.
- First, specific bony structures such as the PSIS, sacral crest, spinous process of L5–S1 and sacral horn are palpated.
- The palpating thumb localizes the portion of the sacrum where there is no muscle attachment (between the erector spinae muscle and the gluteus maximus muscle; Fig. **126**).

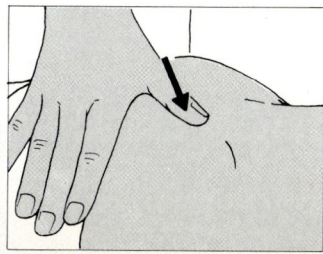

Fig. **126**

Examination Techniques
Sacroiliac Joint and Pelvis
Zones of Irritation S1–S3

Note

- Due to its anatomic position, palpation of these zones is relatively easy, even for the novice.
- Definite differentiation must be made between the individual zones of irritation by way of provocative testing (the so-called "ventralization maneuver" according to Sutter).
- With anterior force directed downward against the sacrum and in the direction of the examination table, the zone of irritation should diminish.
- When the anterior pressure is relieved again, the pain reappears at the previous zone of irritation, often accompanied by a rather stabbing pain (Fig. **127**).

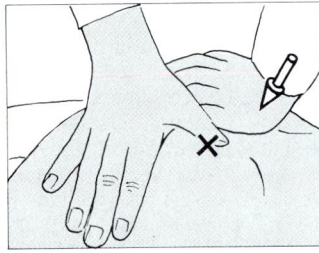

Fig. **127**

Radiologic Diagnosis

- Specific radiologic studies of the spinal region in question become indicated once functional disturbances have been diagnosed clinically or when contraindications for manual therapy need to be determined via these studies.
- This strategy holds especially true for elderly patients when suspecting osteoporosis, primary and secondary tumors, or other bony abnormalities.
- In order to demonstrate segmental hypermobility or hypomobility in the cervical and lumbar spine, functional X-rays are recommended: primarily lateral projections, and occasionally AP projections.

Cervical Spine

- Routine studies before manual treatment include lateral and AP views of the cervical spine.
- After cervical spine trauma, the open-mouth view should be utilized so as to exclude fracture of the dens or injury to the atlanto-axial and atlanto-occipital joints.
- In the case of significant degenerative changes and when suspecting root compression, the oblique views are indicated so as to evaluate the intervertebral foramina as well as the sulci of the spinal nerves.
- When taking functional cervical spine X-rays for flexion and extension movements, the patient should be standing upright with the thoracic spine stabilized.
- Flexion and extension movements should only be introduced by an examiner who has acquired biomechanical experience (Fig. **128**).

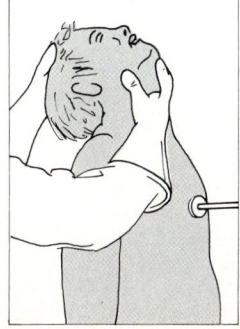
Fig. **128a**

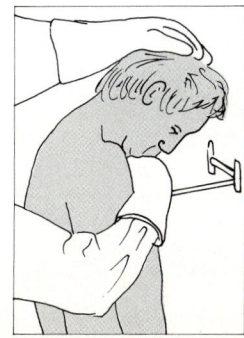
Fig. **128b**

Radiologic Diagnosis

- Measurements are follows: The vertebral bodies are projected over each other in the flexion and extension positions, and a line is drawn along the edge of the X-ray. Segmental range of motion of the vertebrae is recorded in a functional diagram (Figs. **129**, **130**).
- Values are deemed pathologic when they fall outside two standard deviations (either above or below) of those values established for young, healthy adults.

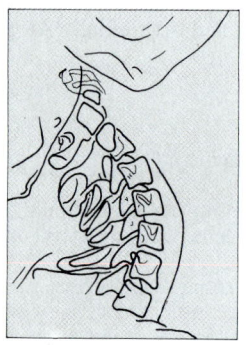
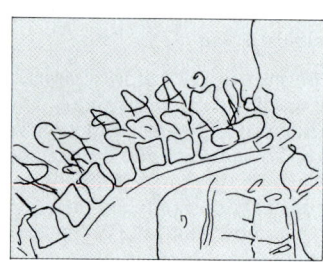

Fig. **129**

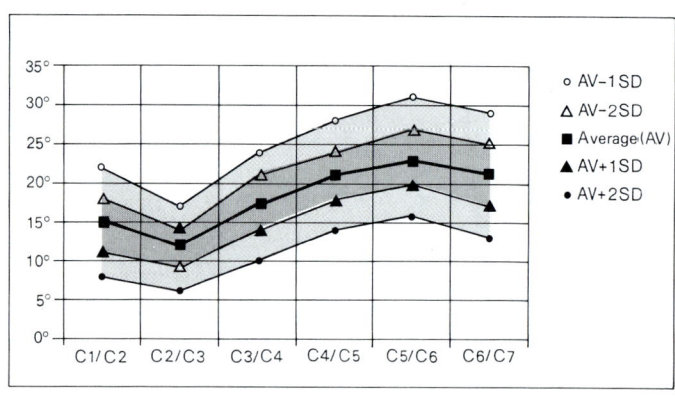

Fig. **130** Functional diagram for flexion and extension in the cervical spine (J. Dvorak et al., 1988)

Radiologic Diagnosis

Thoracic Spine

- The AP view (Fig. **131**) clearly reveals the root of the arch and the spinous processes but less so the articular processes or joint spaces.
- Typically, the head of the rib, in its close anatomic relationship to the disk, can be visualized in addition to the neck of the rib laterally and the tubercle of the rib. The costotransverse joint space is visible in the lower segments.
- Due to its oblique and inferiorly directed arrangement, the tip of the spinous process in the midthoracic spine is projected over the next inferior vertebral body.

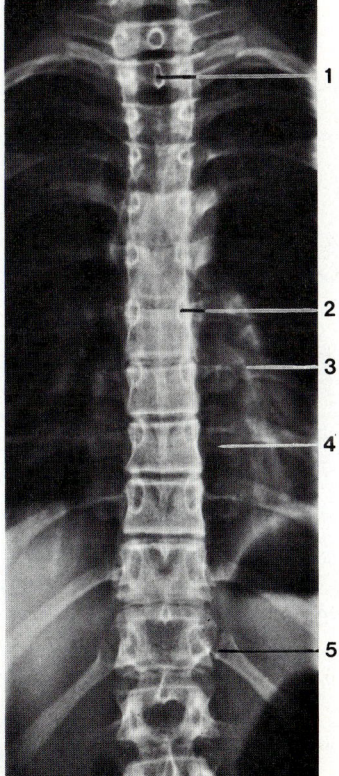

Fig. **131** Radiograph of the thoracic spine, AP view (after L. Lewit); 1) spinous process, 2) root of the arch, 3) rib, 4) transverse process, 5) costotransverse joint

Radiologic Diagnosis

- Positional asymmetries should not be overinterpreted. Vertebral rotation should only be suspected when positional asymmetry is found in addition to an asymmetry in the distance between the root of the arch and the outer margin of the vertebral body.
- The lateral view (Fig. **132**) clearly reveals the shape of the vertebrae and the intervertebral discs as well as the intervertebral foramina, the joint space and the articular processes.
- The ribs are frequently projected over the vertebral arch and the spinous process.
- In the lateral view, abnormal posture, growth abnormalities (e.g., status post Scheuermann's disease, or juvenile kyphosis), and degenerative disk disease can be demonstrated.

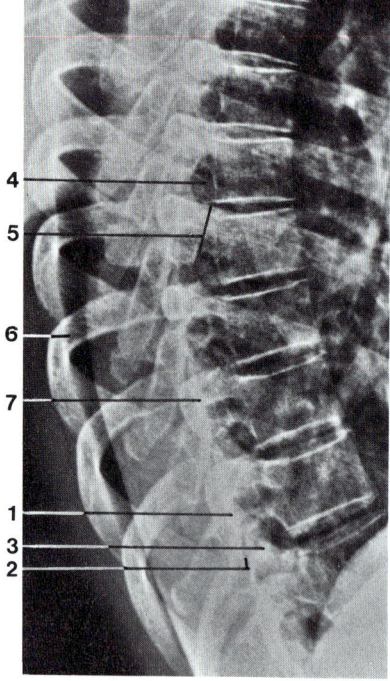

Fig. **132** Radiograph of the thoracic spine, lateral view (after L. Lewit); 1) inferior articular process; 2) joint space; 3) superior articular process; 4) intervertebral foramen; 5) vertebral arch; 6) rib; 7) transverse process

Radiologic Diagnosis

Lumbar Spine and Pelvis

- The plate size commonly used for thorax exposures (35 mm × 43 mm) is actually very well suited to provide an anteroposterior view of both the entire lumbar spine and pelvis, including the symphysis pubis and femoral heads (Fig. **133**). This view, taken with the patient in the standing position, provides more meaningful information than the narrow view of the spine alone or a pelvic view with the patient in the supine position.

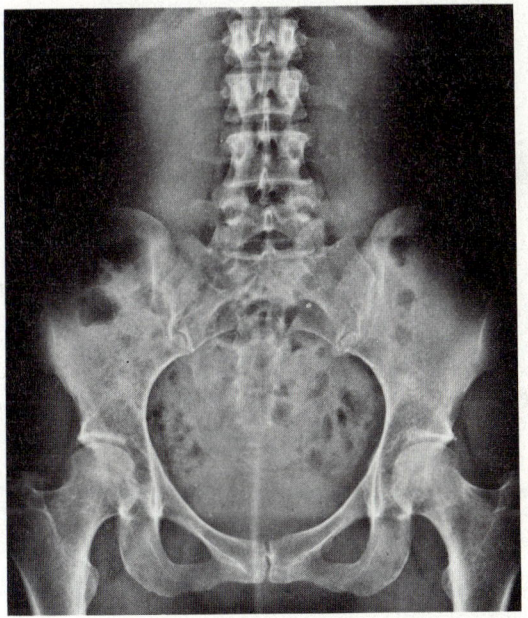

Fig. **133** Lumbar spine and pelvis, AP view. Facet joints at L4–L5 and L5–S1 lie in frontal plane on the right and in sagittal plane on the left

Radiologic Diagnosis

- Pelvic torsions that may cause a functional disturbance in the sacroiliac joint can be recognized by the asymmetric appearance on the radiograph (Fig. **134**). In this view, the examiner evaluates whether the symphysis pubis is level (unilateral elevation of the symphysis) and if there is asymmetry of the obturator foramina, or unilateral hiking of the pelvis crest with the ilium being narrower on one side when compared to the other.

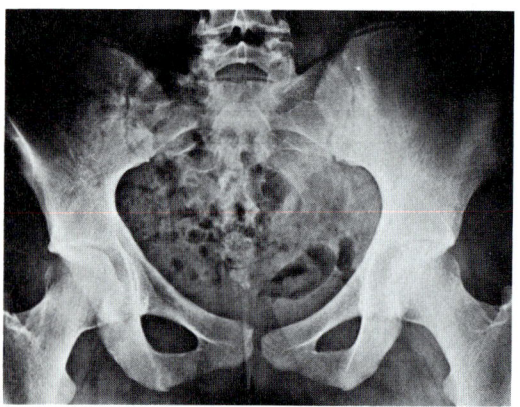

Fig. 134 Pelvic torsion (patient supine). Asymmetric projection of the pelvic halves, superior symphysis, and asymmetric obturator foramen

- This view also allows preliminary interpretation of the hip joint, especially the relationship between the femoral head and neck, the hip socket, and the leg length.
- Whether, and to what extent, a leg-length difference causes changes in the lumbar spine is in part dependent on the position of the lumbar facet joints.
- Between L1 and L3, the facet joints, because their orientation is more in the sagittal plane, can be well visualized on an AP view. In contrast, asymmetries are frequently seen in the facet joints at the L4–L5 level, and in particular the L5–S1 level. Radiographically, these joints appear oriented more in the frontal plane unilaterally. Such changes may then alter the relationship of the loading forces, leading to abnormal movement patterns and thus contributing to asymmetric degenerative changes.

Radiologic Diagnosis

- In the lumbar spine specifically, the shape and positional relationship of the vertebral bodies, the intervertebral disks, and the roots of the vertebral arch are evaluated (Fig. **135**).

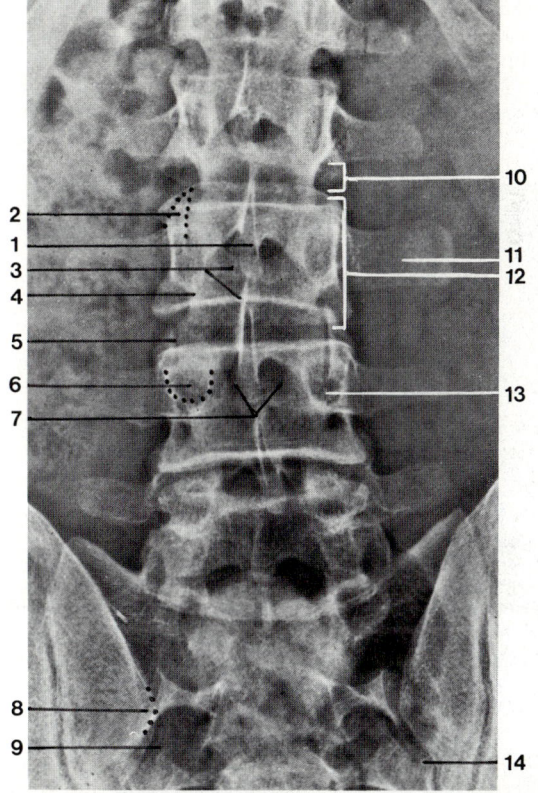

Fig. **135** Radiograph of the lumbar spine, AP view (after L. Lewit); 1) spinous process; 2) upper articular process; 3) vertebral arch; 4) interarticular area; 5) joint space; 6) inferior articular process; 7) spinal cana; 8) posterior inferior iliac spine (PSIS); 9) sacroiliac joint; 10) intervertebral disk; 11) transverse process; 12) vertebral body; 13) vertebral arch; 14) sacroiliac joint

Radiologic Diagnosis

- The lowermost lumbar vertebra has the greatest tendency to reveal an anomaly such as spina bifida occulta (the incomplete union of both laminae to form the spinous process), which is usually of less significance than those unilateral junctional abnormalities, for instance, in which the transverse processes have become unfittingly large. In the latter case, these huge transverse processes may make actual contact with the lateral mass of the sacrum, leading to irritations in that area and subsequently causing sclerosis in the adjoining bony components.
- The lateral view (Fig. **136**) which should, if possible, always include the femoral heads, may demonstrate a pelvic torsion. The pelvic

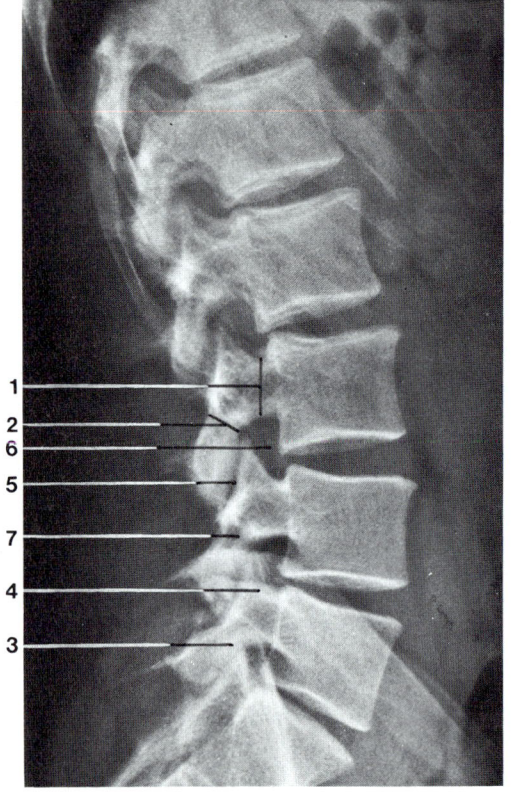

Fig. **136** Lateral view of the lumbar spine, radiograph (after L. Lewit); 1) vertebral arch; 2) interarticular space; 3) inferior articular surface; 4) superior articular surface; 5) joint space; 6) intervertebral foramen; 7) transverse process

Radiologic Diagnosis

crests would then appear as incongruent, and would intersect at the level of the facet joints (Fig. **137**).

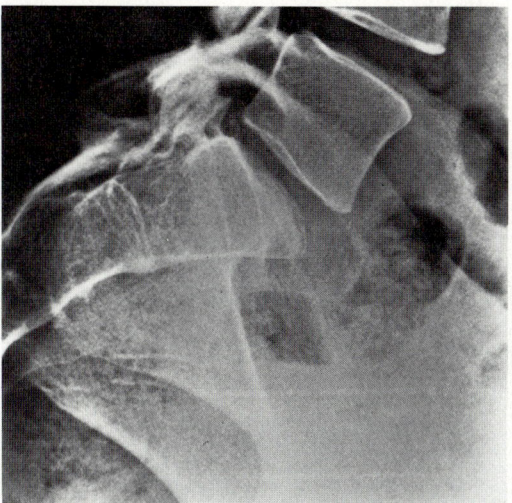

Fig. **137** Lateral view of the lumbosacral junction that may reveal pelvic torsion when the pelvic crests intersect at the level of the facet joints

- The degree of the spinal curvatures in the sagittal plane (i.e., exaggerated versus reversed lordotic curvature in the lumbar spine), along with variations in the sacral base inclination, have been used to define three pelvic types: the arch-type (high assimilation) pelvis, the normal pelvis (block pelvis), and the flat-type pelvis.
- It is also possible to statically differentiate between a real spondylolisthesis with a bony break in the interarticular portion and an anterior or posterior pseudolisthesis with spondyloarthrosis and osteochondrosis.
- For manual therapy, differentiation between instability and osteophytic reaction is of greater significance than the recognition of the mere presence of pelvic type, junctional anomalies, or spondylolisthesis.

Radiologic Diagnosis

- Instability can be detected on a radiograph by so-called traction marks that are due to overstretching of the outermost fibers of the annulus (Figs. **138, 139**). On the radiograph, these appear as horizontal ossifications up to 1 mm in length projecting from the edge of the vertebral body. This is in contrast to the marginal osteophytes that grow towards each other and restrict movement but usually do not cause segmental dysfunction.

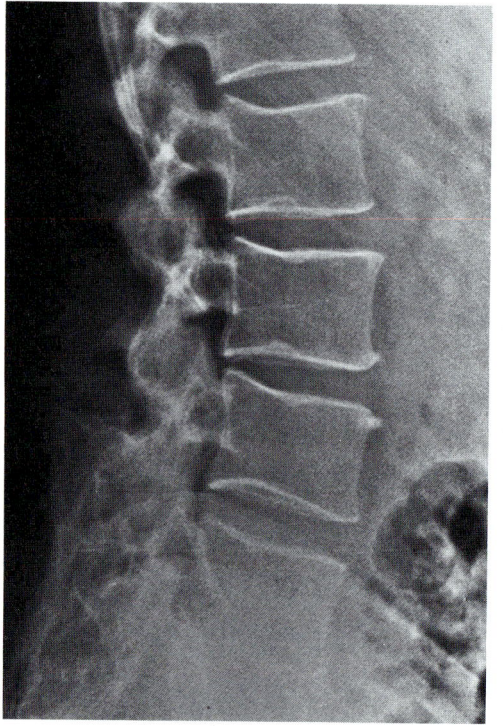

Fig. **138** Lateral view of the lumbar spine with traction marks at the L3–L4 segment

Radiologic Diagnosis

- In contrast, hypermobile spinal segments are frequently associated with segmental dysfunction and require very specific therapy.
- Functional views in extension and flexion may occasionally reveal excessive hypermobility, however, with "normal values" assuming a rather large range.

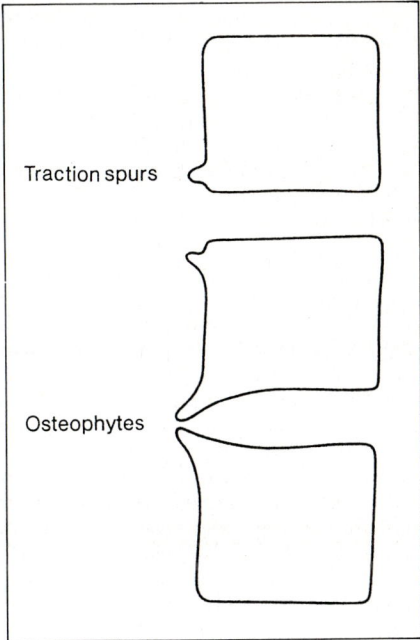

Fig. **139** Instability results in overstretch of the outermost fibers of the annulus fibrosus, leading to horizontal traction marks. Osteophytes grow towards each other, leading to less mobility and greater stabilization where they grow together

Indications, Contraindications, Complications

Indications

- The goal of manual therapy is the restoration of function of the individual spinal segments and/or entire spinal regions as well as the extremity joints.
- If a reversible functional disturbance is suspected (i.e., somatic dysfunction), specific manual therapy can be expected to restore function.
- Acute painful spinal syndromes are rewarding indications for specific manual therapy.
- Even though these syndromes tend to have a rather high percentage of spontaneous recovery, it has been borne out that manual therapy is superior to such conservative treatment as rest, pure pain medication, or only physiotherapeutic management.
- Empirical findings have been supported by controlled studies.
- Patients with chronic and chronic-recurrent spinal syndromes, usually due to degenerative changes such as osteochondrosis and spondyloarthrosis, are candidates for manual therapy, however, treatment results are usually less spectacular.
- Secondary symptoms, including pain, may be positively influenced by manual therapy.
- Treatment of patients with chronic back pain, who as a rule reveal a significant muscular imbalance with shortening and weakening of individual muscle groups, will usually be treated with mobilization techniques without impulse, or muscle techniques, rather than techniques that utilize impulse (i.e., classic thrust techniques).
- Manual treatment of both the extremity joints and the spinal segment plays an important role in pain treatment. These manual techniques induce presynaptic inhibition of pain transmission at the level of the spinal cord, by stimulation of the mechanoreceptor in the periphery. Adequate manual therapy may then prepare the patient for appropriate physical therapy and muscular rehabilitation.
- In the treatment of cervical syndromes, the presence of vertigo requires special attention. It is imperative to exclude other causes for vertigo first (differential diagnosis) before attempting to treat the patient in whom cervical vertigo is diagnosed. Once a diagnosis of cervical vertigo has been made, the use manual therapy may be very favorable.
- An individual listing for specific disorders (i.e., a list of indications) becomes dispensable as long as the guidelines of manual diagnosis have been followed and classic orthopedic and medical examinations have been included wherever indicated.

Indications, Contraindications, Complications
Indications

- In summary, the following clinical situations affecting the musculoskeletal apparatus have been found to be amenable to manual therapy:
  1. Acute, painful functional disturbances in the spinal segments without radicular symptomatology.
  2. Chronic and chronic-recurrent spinal syndromes, accompanied by secondary muscular changes (increased tone; palpable, taut bands) accompanied by muscular imbalance.
  3. Symptomatic treatment of pain in patients with degenerative changes affecting the spinal peripheral joints.

Patient Response to Manual Therapy

- If the patient feels improvement after treatment, the treatment can be repeated until the patient is symptom-free or until the treatment goal has been reached.
- Occasionally, and in particular after mobilization with impulse techniques (thrust techniques), the patient's symptoms can be exacerbated for minutes to hours after treatment but show improvement the day after treatment. In this situation, the treatment regimen should be continued as well. Previous examination of findings should be re-evaluated, however, and should be very well documented.
- If treatment causes progressively worsening symptoms over days, the manipulative treatment regimen should be discontinued. Previous examination findings need to be reviewed and re-evaluated. If additional symptoms become apparent, the patient may need to be referred to a neurologist, rheumatologist, or physiatrist.
- In case of immediate neurologic complications or those that occur after a latency period of hours to days, the patient should be referred to a medical center for further in-depth neurologic evaluation and possible hospitalization. The treatment procedure as well as diagnostic findings must be documented very carefully.

Indications, Contraindications, Complications
Contraindications

- Acute lumbar disk herniation with radicular symptomatology.
- Acute cervical disk herniation with or without radicular symptoms.
- Recent soft-tissue injuries to the cervical spine (4−8 weeks after the accident).
- Vascular vertigo due to vertebral-basilar insufficiency.
- Bony malformations in the spine.
- Spinal cord abnormalities.
- Marked osteoporosis, metabolic abnormalities affecting the bone with an increased tendency to have pathologic fractures.
- Ankylosing spondylitis in the acute inflammatory stage.
- Inflammatory processes affecting the spine in the presence of rheumatoid arthritis.
- Post-traumatic segmental hypermobility.
- Tumors and metastases.
- Complications are actually rare when the guidelines for appropriate manual therapy are followed, including appropriate indication and contraindication. Complications are less likely to occur when the practitioner has greater experience in the various techniques. On the average, out of approximately 400 000 treatments to the cervical spine, one major complication may occur.
- Manual therapy of the thoracic and lumbar spine rarely leads to complications. though there continue to be reports that manipulative intervention causes disk protrusion resulting in radicular symptomatology.

Manual Therapy
Concepts of Manual Therapy

- It is felt that manual therapy stimulates the individual mechanoreceptors.
- Stimulation of the mechanoreceptor presynaptically inhibits pain conduction at the level of the gelatinous substance in the spinal cord.
- The exact mechanisms by which the effects of manual therapy come about, in particular those of the classic thrust techniques (mobilization with impulse), have not been conclusively elucidated. It is conceivable that, in addition to alleviating pain, the treatment techniques release an otherwise dislodged meniscoid (i.e., in the cervical spine) or that specific rotatory techniques displace the nucleus pulposus away from the nerve structures, thereby relieving pressure from the facet joints over the nerve root.
- Restoration of muscle balance plays a paramount role in prevention of pain recurrence in spinal syndromes.
- Stretching of the shortening tonic muscles as well as strengthening of the weak phasic muscles, including appropriate instructions for home training and back school, have become a routine component of manual therapy.

(The following sections on manual therapy are based primarily on the text *Manual Medicine: Therapy* by W. Schneider, J. Dvořák, V. Dvořák and T. Tritschler [Stuttgart: Thieme, 1988].)

Concepts of Manual Therapy
Mobilization without Impulse

Basic Principles

Vertebral Column

- The spinal segments adjoining the restricted spinal segments are carried to their respective barriers (slack is taken up).
- The operator should make bony contact only with those structures that are located outside a zone of irritation.
- Mobilization is to be performed in the pain-free direction.
- The direction of mobilization is determined by the results obtained through provocative testing. Mobilization is done in the direction in which the pain and nociceptive reactions are diminished.
- The duration of the mobilization technique ranges between 3 and 10 seconds.
- Mobilization should not go beyond the anatomic motion barrier.
- Traction may be utilized to treat pain as well.

Extremity Joints

The restricted joint is carried to its present neutral position (resting position).
- The hands are placed as close to the joint as possible, and in most instances the proximal joint partner is fixated, with the distal part being mobilized.
- Mobilization direction is chosen according to the convex or concave rule, leading to greater mobility in that particular joint (Schmidt, Dvořák).
- Traction may be used to help alleviate pain prior to applying these specific mobilization techniques.
- Mobilization of the individual joint should not go beyond the anatomic motion barrier.
- Mobilization without impulse must be performed gently and without inflicting pain on the patient.

Manual Therapy
Concepts of Manual Therapy
Mobilization with Impulse (Classic Thrust)

Basic Principles

Vertebral Column

- In the United States, manipulation is a rather general term referring to any therapeutic procedure in which the hands are used to treat the patent. In Europe, manipulation specifically refers to what is described in the English language (or according to American osteopathic terminology) as "high velocity, low amplitude thrust."
- Slack is taken up in the spinal segments adjoining the restricted joints (the neighboring segments are at their respective barriers).
- Positioning of the patient should not be painful.
- The choice of direction for the mobilization with impulse is determined by the results from provocative testing. Mobilization is effected in the direction in which pain and nociceptive reactions are diminished (Fig. **140**).
- The impulse force should be of sufficient magnitude to introduce movement in the restricted joints but not beyond the anatomic barrier.

Extremity Joints

- The restricted joint is brought to its present neutral position.
- The operator places his hands close to the joint and fixates the proximal joint partner. The impulse is usually introduced perpendicular to the treatment plane.

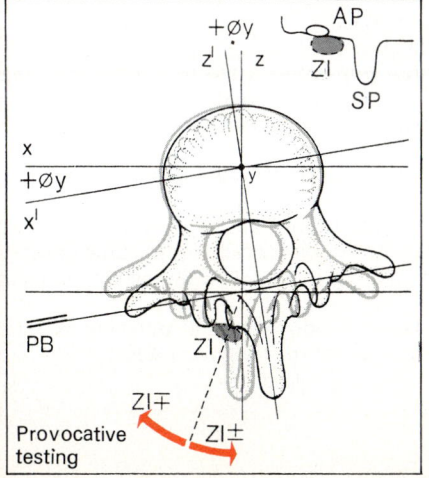

ZI   zone of irritation
SP   spinous process
AP   articular process
PB   pathologic barrier
     (limit of movement)
$z-z' = +\emptyset y$
$x-x' = +\emptyset y$

Fig. **140** Provocative testing for quantitative changes in the zone of irritation.

Manual Therapy
Concepts of Manual Therapy
Neuromuscular Therapy

- Neuromuscular therapy is a form of treatment in which those techniques are utilized that improve mobility and stretch the muscles either by direct muscle action or as a consequence of associated neuromuscular reflex mechanisms.

NMT 1: Mobilization Utilizing Direct Muscle Force of the Agonists

- Starting from the engaged pathologic barrier, the patient effects mobilization by contracting the appropriate agonistic muscles. This brings about movement beyond the pathologic barrier.
- The slack is taken up in the spinal segments adjoining the restricted joint.
- NMT 1 teaches the patient those mobilization techniques he or she can later perform on his or her own (i.e., self-mobilization).

NMT 2: Mobilization Utilizing Postisometric Relaxation of the Antagonists

- If muscle testing reveals shortened tonic muscles, then there will always be diminished associated regional mobility, be it in the spinal areas (Fig. **141a**) or the extremity joints. Isometric contraction of one muscle followed by stretching of that muscle during the postisometric relaxation phase may lengthen it, often restoring its normal length.
- NMT 2 may be most beneficial in cases in which there is a soft endfeel observed while evaluating angular range of motion.

Basic Principles

- The incriminated muscle is brought into to a position of maximal stretch, at which point the patient is requested to optimally contract the muscle isometrically in a direction away from the pathologic motion barrier (Fig. **141b**).
- Then, during the postisometric relaxation phase, the muscle is stretched for about 3–10 seconds (Fig. **141c**).
- Stepwise stretching: starting from this newly gained position, the patient is again requested to isometrically contract the muscle to the maximum, which is then again stretched during the postisometric relaxation phase.
- In most cases, the patient needs to learn a stretching-exercise program that is followed at home on a regular basis.

Manual Therapy
Concepts of Manual Therapy
Neuromuscular Therapy

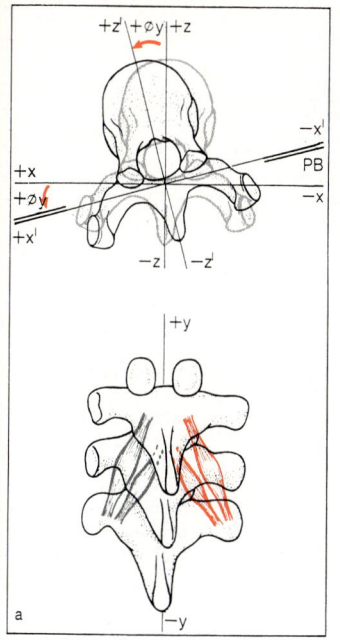
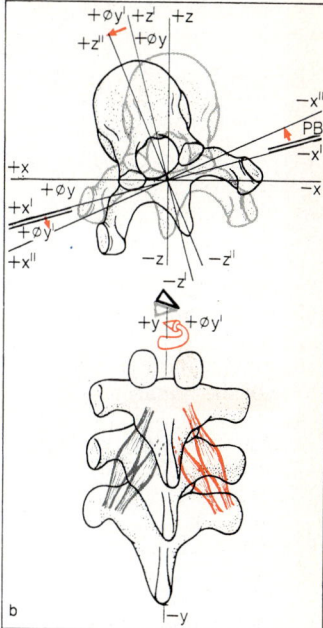

Fig. 141 NMT 2 (i.e., rotation right [– ∅y] is limited by shortening of the right transversospinal muscle system)

a Conflict situation:
 +z−(+z′) = + ∅y
 +x−(+x′) = + ∅y
 Red: shortened rotation antagonist muscles (rotator muscles)
 Gray: rotation agonist muscles (rotator muscles)
 PB: pathologic motion barrier

b Isometric contraction:
 +z′−(+z″) = + ∅y′ } extent of isometric contraction
 +x′−(+x″) = + ∅y′
 Red: shortened antagonist rotator muscles
 Gray: rotation agonist muscles
 PB: pathologic motion barrier
  resistance
  direction of isometric contraction

Manual Therapy
Concepts of Manual Therapy
Neuromuscular Therapy

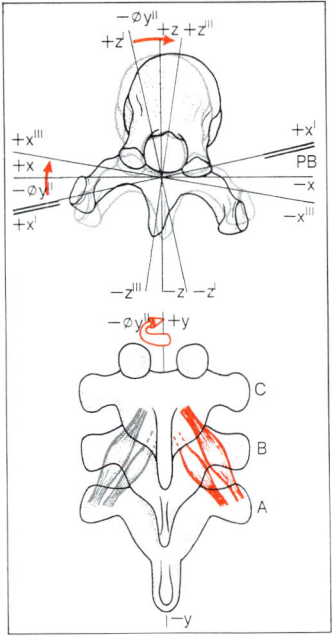

Abb. **141 c**
c Mobilization step:
$+z'-(+z''') = +\emptyset y''$ } gain in mobil-
$+x'-(+x''') = +\emptyset y''$ } ity

Red: rotation agonist muscles (rotator muscles)
Gray: rotation agonist muscles that provide stretch (rotator muscles)
A: fixed vertebra
B, C mobilizing vertebra
PB: pathologic motion barrier
↶ mobilization/stretching direction

NMT 3: Mobilization Utilizing Reciprocal Inhibition of the Antagonists

- Isometric contraction is in the direction of motion restriction. The muscles antagonistic to those muscles that need to be relaxed are isometrically contracted, with the restricted joints being fixated. This is in contrast to NMT 1 in which the spinal segments adjoining the restricted joint are fixated.
- This technique is utilized when isometric contraction of the shortened tonic musculature is painful.

Manual Therapy
Concepts of Manual Therapy
Back School

Back School, Home Exercise Program

- The physician must be convinced of the effectiveness of a home exercise program. The patient must be motivated and ready to fully participate in such a program.
- *Home exercises:* These are based on specific findings of regional restriction so that the patient can mobilize these areas by him- or herself as well as stretch certain muscles and strengthen certain others.
- *Back school:* These are usually run by physical therapists emphasizing physiologic posture, movement, and restoration of muscular balance (10–12 lessons). The physician provides basic information about functional anatomy, biomechanics, and pathology affecting the spine in two 20-minute lectures.
- The back school has proved to be one of the best preventive measures for functional spinal syndromes.

Manual Therapy
Cervical Spine
C0–C1

Treatment

Mobilization without impulse: flexion–extension.

Indication

- Flexion–extension restriction in the upper cervical spinal joint.
- Hard endfeel with pain at the extreme of motion.
- Sublocalized suboccipital pain, possibly radiating towards the occiput.
- Zone of irritation, C0–C1.
- Shortening of the suboccipital muscles.

Treatment Procedure

- Patient sitting.
- Standing at the patient's side, the operator stabilizes the patient's trunk against his or her thigh.
- The atlas is gently fixated at the articular pillars by the operator's thumb and index finger.
- With the other hand placed broadly over the patient's temporal region, the patient's head is cradled in the operator's arm and stabilized against the operator's chest (Fig. **142**).
- Passive mobilization without impulse is introduced by alternatingly moving back and forth between flexion and extension beyond the pathologic barrier.

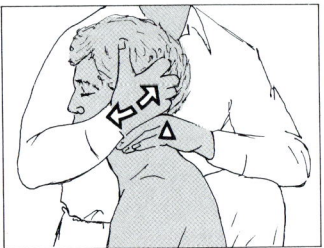

Fig. **142**

Note

- It is important to achieve good stabilization of the head and a gentle fixation of the atlas.

Manual Therapy
Cervical Spine
C0–C4

Treatment

Mobilization without impulse: axial traction.

Indication

- Motion restriction in the upper cervical spine.
- Hard endfeel at the motion barrier, sometimes accompanied by pain.
- Diffuse pain in the neck region. Pain with movement.
- Zones of irritation.
- Shortening of the suboccipital muscles.

Treatment Procedure

- Operator stands behind the sitting patient.
- The operator places both hands flat over the side of the patient's head in the parietal region.
- The forearms fixate the patient's shoulders.
- During exhalation, passive traction is introduced (Fig. **143**).

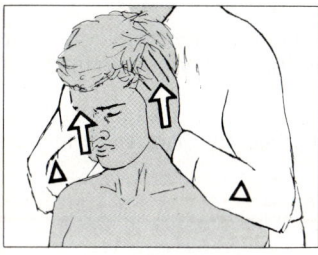

Fig. **143**

Note

- Traction should be synchronized with inhalation and exhalation movement.
- This is a rather gentle treatment with minimal risk.

Manual Therapy
Cervical Spine
C1–C2

Treatment

Mobilization NMT 2, rotation.

Indication

- Rotation restriction in the upper cervical spinal joints.
- Localized suboccipital pain with radiate towards the occiput.
- Zones of irritation C1, C2.
- Shortening of the suboccipital muscles with soft endfeel and occasional pain at the barrier of movement.

Treatment Procedure

- Patient sitting.
- Standing at the patient's side, the operator fixates the patient's trunk against his or her thigh.
- The operator places the thumb and index finger over the articular processes of C2, thereby fixating the vertebra.
- With the other arm, the operator cradles the patient's head and places the small finger over the posterior arch of the atlas.
- The spinal segment in question is carried to its pathologic motion barrier.
- Against equal and opposite operator resistance, the patient is requested to contract isometrically the shortened rotation-antagonist muscles (1; Fig. **144a**).
- During the postisometric relaxation phase, passive rotation to the head is introduced, at which time the shortened muscles are stretched (2; Fig. **144b**).

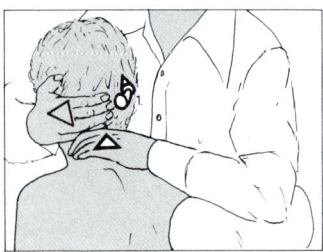
Fig. **144a**

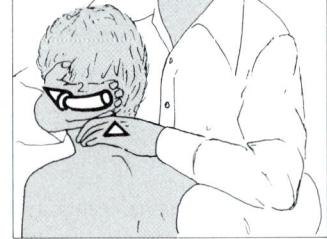
Fig. **144b**

Note

- The individual mobilization advance is rather small.
- Force applied must be carefully dosed in the suboccipital region.

Manual Therapy
Cervical Spine
C2–C6

Treatment

Mobilization with impulse, rotation restriction.

Indication

- Segmental hypomobility.
- Hard endfeel at the motion barrier with pain at the end of movement.
- Localized pain, occasionally shoulder, arm, and neck pain.
- Zones of irritation.

Treatment Procedure

- Operator stands behind the sitting patient.
- The operator places the second metacarpal bone over the vertebra below the spinal segment to be mobilized.
- The small finger of the other hand is placed over the vertebra above the segment to be mobilized in order to stabilize it.
- By turning the patient's head, passive cervical spine rotation is introduced to the motion barrier of the spinal segment involved (localization of the spinal segment in question).
- During exhalation, a rotatory impulse force (thrust) is introduced (Fig. **145**).

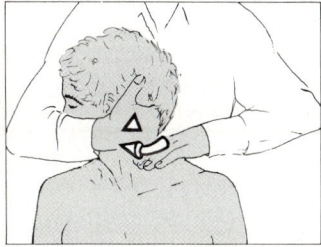

Fig. **145**

Note

- This is the technique of choice for problems in the midcervical spine.
- Make sure that the patient is relaxed.
- This technique should only be applied by an experienced operator.
- If dizziness occurs with positioning, the procedure must be terminated immediately.

Manual Therapy
Cervical Spine
C2–C6

Treatment

Mobilization with impulse, rotation.

Indication

- Segmental motion restriction with hard endfeel.
- Pain at the extreme of movement (motion barrier).
- Pain in the neck, localized or occasionally radiating to the shoulder and area between the shoulder blades.
- Zones of irritation, C2–C6.

Treatment Procedure

- Patient sitting.
- The operator stands at the patient's side.
- The middle finger through which the impulse force is introduced is placed over the articular pillar of the vertebra in question.
- The other hand fixates the patient's head at the parietal region.
- Passive lateral side-bending is introduced to the neck so as to guide the restricted segment to its pathologic motion barrier.
- Following along the inclination of the facet joints, the impulse (thrust) is introduced through the transverse process in an anterior and superior direction (Fig. **146**).

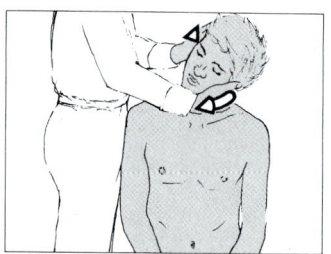

Fig. **146**

Note

- This technique requires very good localization and exact positioning at the motion barrier.
- The impulse is introduced during exhalation.
- The rotation movement introduced with the impulse should be rather small.
- In the hands of an experienced practitioner, this becomes a gentle and very efficient technique.

Manual Therapy
Cervical Spine
C2–C7

Treatment

Mobilization NMT 2, rotation restriction.

Indication

- Segmental rotation restriction with soft endfeel. Pain at the motion barrier.
- Very frequently, the patient presents with chronic pain in the neck region, which may occasionally radiate towards the occiput or shoulder area.
- Zones of irritation.
- There may be shortening of the deep rotator muscles (postural muscles such as the rotatores muscles, multifidus muscle, semispinalis muscle) and the descending portion of the trapezius muscle as well as the levator scapulae muscle.

Treatment Procedure

- Patient sitting.
- The operator, standing at the patient's side, stabilizes the patient's trunk against his or her thigh.
- The inferior partner of the spinal segment that is to be treated is fixated by the operator's thumb and index finger placed gently over the articular processes.
- The other hand cradles the patient's head as well as the upper cervical spinal joints.
- By rotating the head only so far, the operator localizes exactly the segment in question and finally guides it to its pathologic barrier.
- The patient is then requested to isometrically contract the shortened rotation-antagonist muscles by pushing in the opposite direction (away from the pathologic barrier; 1). The operator provides equal but opposite resistive force with the fixating hand (Fig. **147a**).
- During the postisometric relaxation phase, the operator introduces passive rotation mobilization beyond the pathologic barrier with simultaneous stretching of the shortened muscles (2; Fig. **147b**).

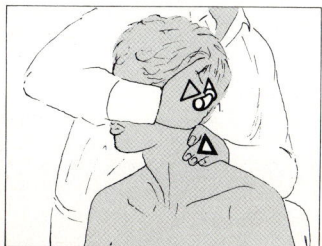

Fig. **147a**

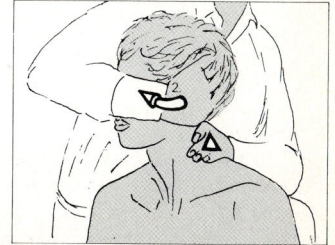

Fig. **147b**

143

Manual Therapy
Cervical Spine
C2–C7

Note

- *Important:* Gentle fixation of the cervical spine is of the utmost importance.
- During the isometric contraction, the patient is also requested to look in the same direction as the contraction.
- During the mobilization phase, the patient looks in the same direction as the stretching.

Manual Therapy
Cervical Spine
C2–C6

Treatment

Mobilization with impulse, rotation restriction.

Indication

- Segmental motion restriction with hard endfeel.
- Pain at the motion barrier.
- Localized pain in the midcervical spine, pain occasionally radiating through the shoulder regions.
- Zones of irritation.

Treatment Procedure

- Operator stands behind the sitting patient.
- With the second metacarpal bone and thumb, the operator fixates gently the inferior vertebra of the restricted spinal segment.
- The small finger and hypothenar of the other hand (impulse-inducing hand) fixates the articular pillar of the superior vertebra of the restricted movement.
- By introducing passive rotation to both the head and the cervical spine, the operator localizes the pathologic motion barrier.
- Subsequently, a rotatory mobilizing impulse (thrust) is introduced (Fig. **148**).

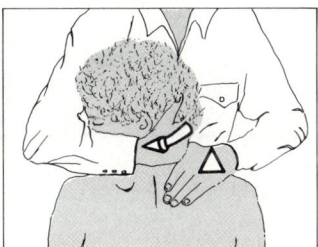

Fig. **148**

Note

- The impulse force is introduced during exhalation; the patient should be totally relaxed.
- *Important:* Positioning at the pathologic motion barrier of the restricted motion segment must be exact.
- In the hands of an experienced operator, this technique is very efficient.

Manual Therapy
Cervicothoracic Junction
C6–T3

Treatment

Mobilization with impulse, rotation.

Indication

- Rotation restriction with hard endfeel and pain at the motion barrier.
- Localized pain in the cervicothoracic region, occasionally radiating to the shoulder region and the area between the shoulder blades.
- Zones of irritation.

Treatment Procedure

- Patient is sitting with the thoracic kyphosis somewhat exaggerated and the cervical spine flexed. Operator stands behind the patient.
- The thumb of the mobilizing hand is placed over the lateral portion of the spinous process of the restricted vertebra.
- With the other hand, the operator introduces passive cervical spine rotation through the patient's head. The spinal segment is carried to its pathologic motion barrier.
- An impulse force in the opposite direction of cervical spine rotation is applied against the spinous process (Fig. **149**).

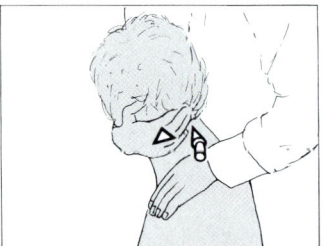

Fig. **149**

Note

- This technique requires rather strong forces, and the patient may report discomfort early on, even during the positioning phase.
- The impulse hand must avoid compression of the lateral neck triangle.

Manual Therapy
Cervicothoracic Junction
C6–T3

Treatment

Mobilization with impulse, rotation and side-bending restriction.

Indication

- Motion restriction of the cervicothoracic junction.
- Hard endfeel with pain at the motion barrier.
- Diffuse and radiating pain in the neck and arm region.
- Zones of irritation.

Treatment Procedure

- Patient is prone.
- The thoracic spine and cervical spine are somewhat flexed.
- The operator, standing at the side of the patient, introduces maximal passive side-bending and rotation of the cervical spine by moving the patient's head.
- Subsequently, the operator places one hand over the patient's head so as to fixate it against the table.
- The mobilizing hand is placed broadly over the shoulder; the arms are crossed.
- During exhalation, the operator introduces a laterally and inferiorly directed impulse force through the hand placed over the shoulder (Fig. **150**).

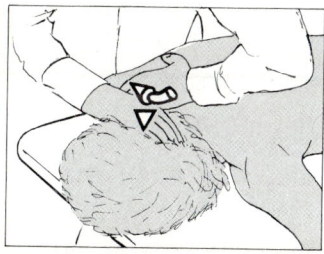

Fig. **150**

Note

- This is a rather nonspecific mobilization technique for the cervicothoracic junction.
- It is imperative to position the patient very gently.

Manual Therapy
Thoracic Spine
T3–T10

Treatment

Mobilization with impulse, traction.

Indication

- Motion restriction in the thoracic spine.
- Localized pain in the thoracic area; pain may occasionally radiate along the ribs in a beltlike distribution.
- Zones of irritation.

Treatment Procedure

- Patient is prone.
- The thoracic kyphosis is exaggerated by positioning such that the apex is localized to the same region of the spinal area that is to be mobilized.
- The operator, standing at the patient's side, places both hands broadly (thenar eminences) over the transverse processes of the segments to be mobilized.
- Simultaneously, both hands effect an impulse against the respective transverse processes with the direction being superior and slightly anterior (Fig. **151**).

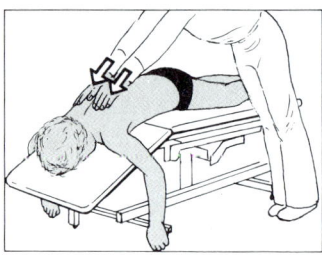

Fig. **151**

Note

- This is a rather efficient, yet nonspecific, manipulation technique.
- *Important:* Impulse force is introduced during exhalation.

Manual Therapy
Thoracic Spine
T3–T10

Treatment

Mobilization with impulse, rotation restriction.

Indication

- Motion restriction in the thoracic spine with hard endfeel.
- Localized pain in the midthoracic spine.
- Pain may be radiating in the thoracic spine along the ribs.
- Zones of irritation.

Treatment Procedure

- Patient is prone.
- The patient's thoracic kyphosis is exaggerated by positioning such that the apex is identical to the segment to be mobilized.
- The operator stands at the patient's side.
- The operator rests his or her crossed hands over the thoracic spine.
- Both pisiform bones are placed with good bony contact over the neighboring transverse processes.
- The operator then introduces an impulse force directed against the transverse processes in an inferior direction (in the direction of the examination table) (Fig. **152**).

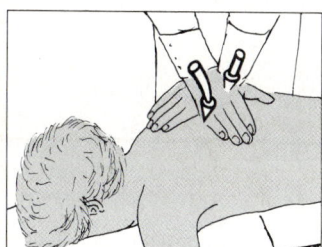

Fig. **152**

Note

- The impulse force must be introduced during exhalation (small resistance).
- This is an efficient and very specific mobilization technique and representative of the classic thrust techniques.

Manual Therapy
Thoracic Spine
T3–T10

Treatment

Mobilization without impulse, rotation.

Indication

- Rotation restriction in the midthoracic spine.
- Pain at the extreme (barrier) of motion.
- Localized pain.
- Zones of irritation.

Treatment Procedure

- Patient sits astride the examination table.
- The operator, standing at the patient's side, reaches around the patient in front and places the hand across the opposite shoulder.
- With the other thumb placed over the spinous process of the vertebra that is to be mobilized, the operator is able to fixate this vertebra.
- Subsequently, the operator introduces passive rotation to the thoracic spine, gently moving beyond the motion barrier and mobilizing the restricted area.
- The thumb provides resistance in the opposite direction (Fig. 153).

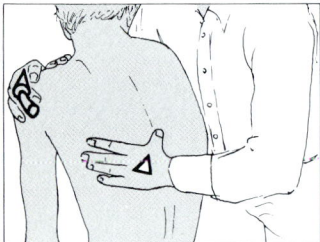

Fig. 153

Manual Therapy
Thoracic Spine
T6–T12

Treatment

Mobilization with impulse, rotation.

Indication

- Segmental motion restriction.
- Hard endfeel with pain at the extreme (barrier) of motion.
- Localized pain with occasionally may radiate towards the ribs.
- Zones of irritation.

Treatment Procedure

- Patient sits astride the examination table.
- The operator, standing at the patient's side, reaches around the patient so as to stabilize both shoulders in front.
- The patient may cross his or her hands in the neck.
- The pisiform bone of the mobilizing hand is placed over the transverse process of the vertebra to be mobilized.
- Subsequently, the operator introduces rotation to the thoracic spine from above until the restricted segment is engaged at its pathologic barrier.
- A short rotatory impulse is effected against the transverse process (Fig. **154**).

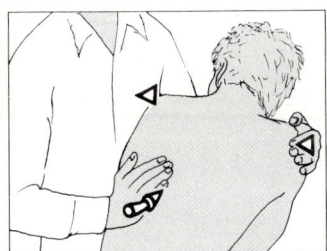

Fig. **154**

Note

- The impulse force should be introduced during exhalation.
- This is a gentle yet efficient technique.

Manual Therapy
Ribs
Rib I

Treatment

Mobilization without impulse.

Indication

- Rib I motion restriction during exhalation (exhalation restriction).
- Pain with movement in the supraclavicular region. Nocturnal paresthesias affecting the arm may occur.
- Zone of irritation at rib I.
- Shortening of the scalene muscles.

Treatment Procedure

- Patient sitting.
- The operator, standing behind the patient, stabilizes with his or her thigh and elbow the shoulder on the side opposite to that of the rib in guestion. With the thumb at the neck, the mobilizing index finger carefully palpates the first rib.
- With the other hand, the operator introduces side-bending of the head and the cervical spine towards the side of the rib to be mobilized (Fig. **155**).
- Passive mobilization in an inferior and medial direction during exhalation.

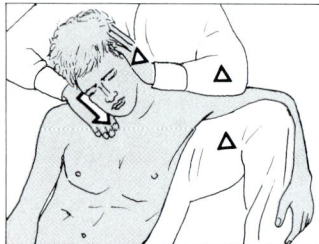

Fig. **155**

Note

- The first rib must be palpated very gently and carefully. Too forceful a pressure may cause paresthesias in the arm.

Manual Therapy
Ribs
Ribs VI–XII

Treatment

Mobilization without impulse.

Indication

- Rib motion restriction.
- Localized stabbing pain, often associated with respiratory movement.
- Pain may also radiate along the ribs in a beltlike manner.
- Zones of irritation at the ribs.

Treatment Procedure

- Patient is prone.
- The operator fixates the rib to be mobilized at the costal angle with his or her pisiform bone.
- The other hand is placed over the anterior iliac spine.
- The involved rib is passively by the operator's rotating the patient's pelvis and lumbar spine to the level of the involved rib (rotation is away from the examination table) (Fig. **156**).

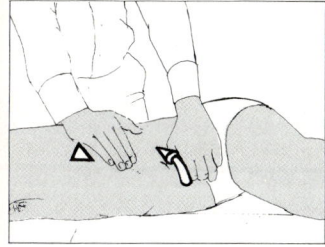

Fig. **156**

Note

- This is a gentle and efficient mobilization technique for the lower ribs.

Ribs
Ribs III–X

Treatment

Mobilization with impulse.

Indication

- Rib motion restriction.
- Pain is posterior and often associated with respiratory movement.
- The pain may also course along the involved ribs radiating to the sternum.
- Zone of irritation at the ribs.

Treatment Procedure

- Patient is prone.
- The thoracic kyphosis is somewhat exaggerated (by flexing the patient's spine).
- The operator places his or her thenar eminence broadly over the costal angle of the involved rib.
- The thenar eminence of the other hand is placed against the spinous process of the vertebra that corresponds to the restricted vertebra.
- An impulse force is effected against the rib in an anterior and inferior direction (following the course of the rib; Fig. **157**).

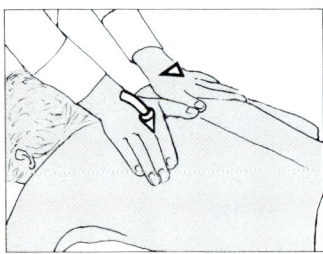

Fig. **157**

Note

- The impulse force is introduced during exhalation.
- *Important:* Good bony contact must be made with the rib to be mobilized.
- This is a rather efficient mobilization technique.

Manual Therapy
Lumbar Spine
L1–L5

Treatment

Mobilization without impulse, rotation.

Indication

- Rotation restriction.
- Hard endfeel with pain at the extreme (barrier) of motion. Pain may be localized or diffused in the lumbar spine and may also occasionally radiate in a beltlike manner.
- Zones of irritation.

Treatment Procedure

- Patient in side-lying position.
- The leg that is in direct contact with the examination table is extended, whereas the upper leg is flexed at the hip and knee joint.
- The patient places one hand under his or her head.
- The operator standing at the patient's side places one index and middle finger over the spinous process of the vertebra to be mobilized. To be exact, specific location is on the side of the spinous process that faces the table (1; Fig. **158a**).
- With his other hand, the operator fixates the superior vertebral partner of the restricted segment by placing the fingertips of the index finger or the thenar eminence over the spinous process, specifically the portion that is pointing away from the table (2).
- The thoracic and lumbar spine are rotated by the operator so as to localize exactly the segment to be mobilized and engage it at its pathologic barrier.
- The operator introduces direct traction to the inferior spinous process, thereby effecting passive rotation-mobilization beyond the pathologic motion barrier (Fig. **158b**).

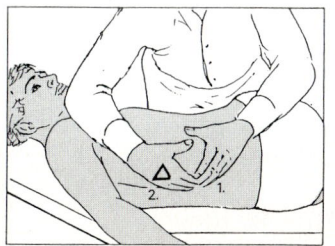

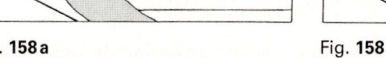

Fig. **158a**   Fig. **158b**

Note

- The patient's head should be rotated in the opposite direction as far as possible.

Manual Therapy
Lumbar Spine
L1–L5

Treatment

Mobilization without impulse, NMT 2, rotation.

Indication

- Segmental rotation motion restriction with soft endfeel due to shortening of the deep rotator muscles in the lumbar spine (rotatores muscles, multifidus and semispinalis muscles), and possibly involvement of the quadratus lumborum muscle.
- Localized pain which may also radiate to the side in a beltlike manner.

Treatment Procedure

- Patient in side-lying position.
- By rotating the thoracic and lumbar spine, the operator engages the pathologic barrier of the spinal segment to be mobilized.
- In the next step, the patient is requested to contract isometrically the shortened muscles away from the motion barrier (1; Fig. **159a**).
- Subsequently, during the isometric relaxation phase and to stretch the shortened muscles as well, mobilization is introduced to the segment beyond the pathologic barrier (2; Fig. **159b**).

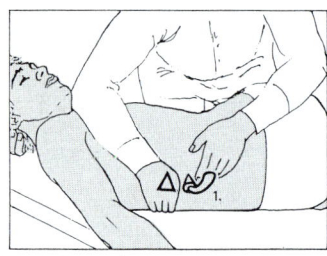
Fig. **159a**

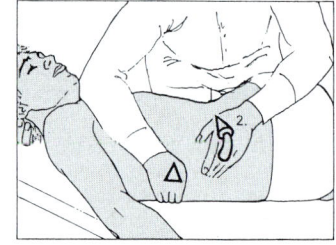
Fig. **159b**

Note

- Isometric contraction should occur during inhalation.
- Stretching and mobilization occurs during exhalation.

Manual Therapy
Lumbar Spine
L1–L5

Treatment

Mobilization with impulse, rotation.

Indication

- Segmental original rotation motion restriction.
- Hard endfeel with pain at the extreme (barrier) of motion.
- Localized and/or radiating pain along the spine or, distributed in a beltlike manner, in the buttocks region or the legs.
- Zones of irritation.

Procedure

- Patient is in the side-lying position, close to the edge of the examination table.
- The operator, standing at the patient's side, grasps the patient's lower arm so as to draw the shoulder closer towards him- or herself.
- There the thoracic and lumbar spine are rotated by the operator until the pathologic barrier of the spinal segment in question is localized and engaged.
- Once in this position, the operator stabilizes the rotated shoulder against the examination table.
- Subsequently, the leg that is away from the table is flexed at the hip and knee joints.
- After the operator has placed his or her own knee against the lateral portion of the patient's knee, he or she is able to indirectly induce passive rotation to the patient's pelvis in the opposite direction.
- The mobilizing hand is placed flat over the lumbar spine and the upper portion of the sacrum, while the forearm rests on the patient's buttocks.
- The operator then places further pressure against the opposite shoulder as well as the patient's knee so as to increase tension and engage the segment at its motion barrier.
- With the spine engaged in this manner, an impulse force is introduced through the hand placed at the lumbar spine; the direction is anterior and inferior (Fig. **160**).

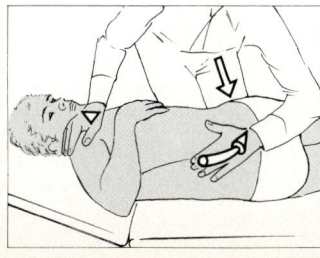

Fig. **160**

Manual Therapy
Lumbar Spine
L1–L5

Note

- The impulse force is introduced during exhalation.
- Positioning should be very gentle and not too time consuming.
- If the patient cannot totally relax, the technique should not be employed.
- If the patient has hip joint problems, he or she may be able to assume the necessary position for set-up of this technique.
- This is a rather nonspecific treatment technique for the lumbar spine.

Manual Therapy
Lumbar Spine
L1–L5

Treatment

Mobilization with impulse, rotation.

Indication

- Segmental rotation restriction.
- Hard endfeel with pain at the extreme (barrier) of motion.
- Localized pain or pain radiating to the gluteal regions and/or the legs.
- Zones of irritation.

Treatment Procedure

- Patient in side-lying position, near the edge of the examination table.
- Positioning and engagement of the spinal segment at the pathologic motion barrier is identical to that for the mobilization technique without impulse previously described for the same area.
- The middle finger and index finger of the mobilizing hand are placed together over the spinous process of the incriminated vertebra.
- During the next step, a short, intensive, rotatory impulse force is introduced against the spinous process of the segment to be mobilized in an anterior and superior direction following rotation (Fig. **161**).

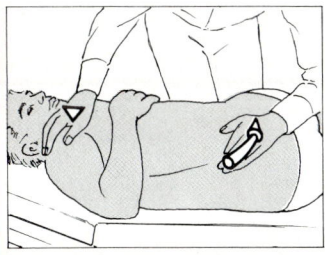

Fig. **161**

Note

- This is a specific and well-localized treatment technique.
- It is imperative to position and engage the spinal segment that is to be mobilized very carefully.

Manual Therapy
Lumbar Spine
L2–L5

Treatment

Mobilization without impulse; flexion and extension.

Indication

- Flexion and extension restriction in the lumbar spine.
- Hard endfeel with pain at the extreme (barrier) of movement.
- Zones of irritation.
- Shortening of the longissimus lumborum muscle.

Treatment Procedure

- Patient in side-lying position, close to the edge of the examination table. The hip and knee joints of both legs are flexed.
- The operator, facing the patient's trunk, leans over him.
- One hand is placed over the spinous process of the superior partner of the restricted spinal segment.
- While fixating the patient's sacrum with his arm, the hand of the same arm palpates the spinous process of the lower partner of the segment in question.
- The operator introduces passive mobilization by enhancing lumbar flexion while simultaneously introducing distraction directed towards the spinous process of the lower vertebra (Fig. **162**).

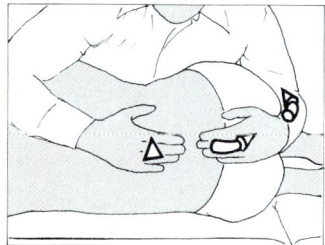

Fig. **162**

Note

- When applied carefully, this may be a good technique in acute, painful syndromes.

Manual Therapy
Sacroiliac Joint

Treatment

Mobilization without impulse, anterior motion restriction (ventralization).

Indication

- Sacroiliac joint (SIJ) motion restriction.
- Acute localized or chronic pain radiating to the gluteal area in a beltlike distribution.
- Zones of irritation.

Treatment Procedure

- Patient is prone.
- The operator places his or her hand over the half of the sacrum that faces the restricted SIJ.
  Through the assistance of the other hand, an anteriorly directed pressure is introduced so as to perform passive sacrum mobilization (Fig. **163**).

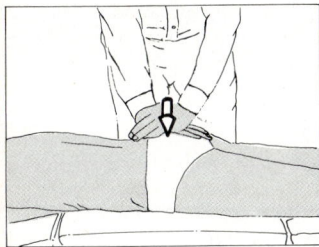

Fig. **163**

Manual Therapy

Sacroiliac Joint

Treatment

Mobilization without impulse, NMT 1.

Indication

- Sacroiliac joint (SIJ) motion restriction.
- Acute localized pain.
- Pain may be chronic and in beltlike manner radiating to the gluteal region.

Treatment Procedure

- Patient is prone.
- One hand is placed over the half of the sacrum that faces the restricted SIJ. The other hand is utilized for support of stabilization.
- With the sacrum stabilized, the patient is requested to lift his or her pelvis off the table on the restricted side (the hip joint is slightly extended, the leg straight; Fig. **164**).

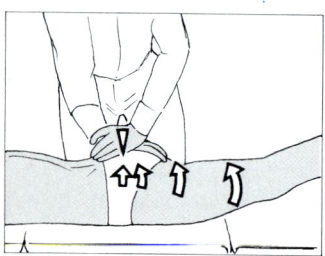

Fig. **164**

Note

- This mobilization procedure is repeated in multiple steps.

Manual Therapy
Sacroiliac Joint

Treatment

Mobilization with impulse.

Indication

- Sacroiliac joint (SIJ) motion restriction.
- Acute, localized deep back pain.
- Pain may also be chronic and diffuse in distribution, sometimes radiating towards the buttocks, either unilaterally or bilaterally.
- Zones of irritation at the sacrum.

Treatment Procedure

- Patient in side-lying position, lying on the side opposite the restricted SIJ, close to the edge of the examination table.
- The patient flexes the leg that is not in contact with the examination table at both the hip and knee joints.
- The operator, standing at the patient's side, rotates the upper shoulder away, thus introducing rotation to the thoracic spine and lumbar spine.
- The patient is stabilized in this position by the operator's fixating the shoulder against the examination table. The mobilizing hand is placed over the patient's pelvis, to which the mobilizing forces will be introduced.
- Slack is taken up by the operator rotating the shoulder further away while simultaneously guiding the patient's knees with his or her own knee.
- The impulse is effected through the patient's pelvis and is directed anterior and inferiorly (Fig. **165**).

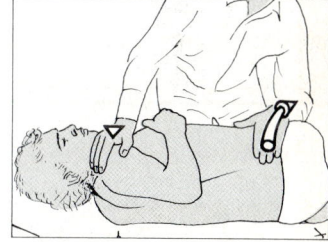

Fig. **165**

Note

- This technique should not be utilized when the patient suffers from hip problems that would prevent adequate positioning.
- The impulse force is effected during the exhalation phase.
- A shortened piriform muscle may impede appropriate positioning, in which case the muscle should be stretched prior to engaging this technique.

Manual Therapy
Sacroiliac Joint

Treatment

Mobilization with impulse.

Indication

- Sacroiliac joint (SIJ) motion restriction.
- The pain can be either localized or diffuse and is deep in the lower back. Pain may also occasionally radiate towards the buttocks and the posterior thigh.
- Zones of irritation, S2, S1 over the sacrum (correlating with provocative testing).

Treatment Procedure

- Patient in side-lying position, lying on the side of the restricted SIJ, close to the edge of the examination table.
- The operator, standing at the patient's side, grasps the patient's distal forearm and pulls the patient's shoulder towards him- or herself.
- The operator then rotates the shoulder as far as possible and stabilizes it in this position against the examination table.
- The patient flexes the leg away from the table at both hip and knee joints.
- The operator places his or her knee over the lateral aspect of the patient's flexed knee for further stabilization.
- The operator places the hypothenar eminence of the mobilizing hand over the half of the sacrum that points in the direction of the table. The impulse is directed anteriorly (Fig. **166**).

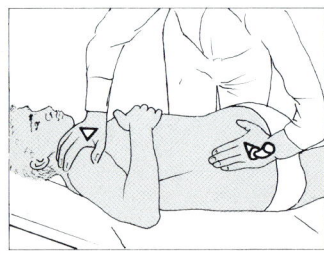

Fig. **166**

Note

- The impulse force is introduced during exhalation.
- A shortened piriform muscle may impede adequate positioning.
- If the patient has any hip problems, this technique should not be engaged.

Manual Therapy
Sacroiliac Joint

Treatment

Mobilization with impulse.

Indication

- Sacroiliac joint (SIJ) motion restriction.
- Localized pain or chronic and deep pain in the lower back with radiation towards the buttocks region, occasionally to the posterior thigh.
- Zone of irritation, S3 (according to provocative testing).

Treatment Procedure

- Patient in side-lying position, close to the edge of the examination table.
- The restricted SIJ is on the side on the table.
- Positioning is identical to that listed for the mobilization technique.
- The operator places the hypothenar eminence of the mobilizing hand over the half of the sacrum on the same side as the restriction.
- At the same time, the hand and forearm are placed broadly over the sacrum.
- Slack is taken out in the SIJ to be mobilized. The patient's opposite shoulder is rotated away, and by monitoring the patient's knees with his or her own knee, the operator prepares the patient such that a thrusting can be effected next.
- The impulse occurs in an inferior and anterior direction (Fig. **167**).

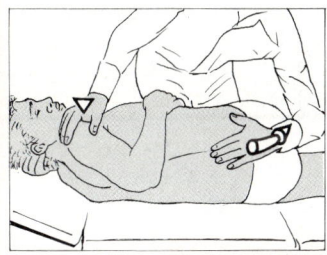

Fig. **167**

Note

- The impulse force is introduced during the exhalation phase.
- Hip pain may become prominent with positioning. This may indicate that excessive rotation has been introduced to the thoracic/lumbar spine.
- A shortened piriform muscle may make positioning more difficult.
- If it is difficult to stabilize and position the hip joint through the flexed leg, it may be due to arthrosis of the hip.

Manual Therapy
Pectoralis major Muscles

Treatment

Stretching, NMT 2.

Indication

- Diminished arm abduction and external rotation.
- Soft endfeel due to shortening of the pectoralis major muscle.
- Pain which may be present in the axilla at the end of arm abduction and external rotation.
- The insertions at the ribs are quite tender to palpation (insertion tendinoses).

Treatment Procedure

- Patient is supine, close to the edge of the examination table. The patient's arm is passively abducted and elevated.
- With his other hand, the operator fixates the patient's thorax at the sternum.
- The patient is requested to contract isometrically the pectoralis major muscle (1). The operator provides an equal but opposite resistant force to the patient's arm.
- During the postisometric relaxation phase, the arm is passively abducted, with additional slight traction (2; Fig. **168**).

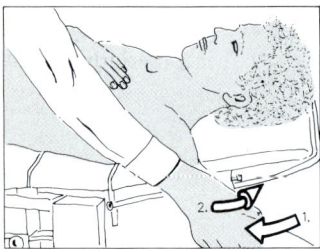

Fig. **168**

Note

- Before applying these techniques, painful changes affecting the humeroscapular joint must be excluded.

Manual Therapy
Trapezius Muscle, Descending Portion

Treatment

Stretching, NMT 2.

Indication

- Gross side-bending restriction and/or rotation restriction in the cervical spine.
- Soft endfeel with pain at the extreme (barrier) of motion.
- Acute local pain.
- Chronic pain of diffuse distribution in the neck region; pain radiating towards the occiput; pain in the shoulder and arm as well as in the interscapular region.

Treatment Procedure

- Patient sitting. The operator, standing behind the patient, stabilizes the patient's shoulder with his forearm on the side that is shortened.
- With his other hand and arm, the operator cradles the patient's head and introduces passive side-bending to the cervical spine. Depending on the course of the shortened muscles that need to be stretched, rotation is introduced to either the same or opposite sides.
- The patient is requested to contract isometrically the shortened muscle for approximately 7–10 seconds (1; the operator's forearm rests on the patient's shoulder).
- During the postisometric relaxation phase, the muscle is passively stretched by mobilizing the shoulder girdle inferiorly and laterally (2; Fig. **169**).

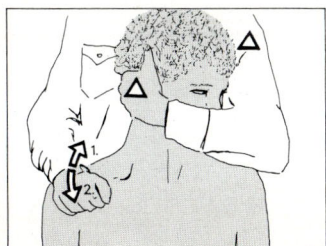

Fig. **169**

Note

- This technique requires several repetitions.
- Isometric contraction should occur during inhalation.
- Stretching should occur during exhalation.

Manual Therapy
Levator scapulae Muscle

Treatment

Stretching, NMT 2.

Indication

- Flexion restriction and/or rotation restriction in the cervical spine.
- Soft endfeel with pain at the extreme (barrier) of motion. The insertions at the border of the shoulder blade are tender.
- Pain in the neck region may be recurrent or chronic, occasionally radiating towards the occiput or the region between the shoulder blades.

Treatment Procedure

- Patient sitting. The operator, standing behind the patient, places the thumb of one hand flat over the spine of the shoulder blade. The other hand is then placed flat over the patient's head, so as to introduce passive cervical spine flexion with slight side-bending and rotation to the opposite side.
- The patient is requested to contract isometrically the shortened levator scapulae muscle against equal but opposite resistance (effectively, the patient attempts to extend the cervical spine against resistance for approximately 7–10 seconds).
- During the postisometric relaxation phase, the muscle is passively stretched by the operator as he introduces further passive cervical spine flexion and rotation to the opposite side (2; Fig. **170**).

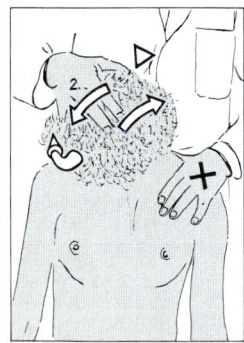

Fig. **170**

Note

- Isometric contractions should occur during inhalation.
- Stretching should be done during the exhalation phase.
- This technique is repeated several times.

Manual Therapy
Sternocleidomastoid Muscle

Treatment

Stretching, NMT 2.

Indication

- Motion restriction of side-bending and rotation in the cervical spine.
- Soft endfeel with pain at the extreme of movement.
- Painful muscle insertions at the clavicle and mastoid process.
- Chronic neck pain, occasionally radiating towards the occiput and/or supraclavicular region.

Treatment Procedure

- Patient sitting with back to the operator.
- The operator places one thumb against the clavicle, thus stabilizing this area (1).
- With his other hand, the operator introduces side-bending to the opposite side and rotation to the same side by moving the patient's head (2).
- The patient is then requested to contract isometrically the shortened sternocleidomastoid muscle against equal but opposite resistance (the head is held stationary by the operator, thus resisting this movement). Overall contraction duration is 7–10 seconds (3; Fig. **171**).
- During the postisometric relaxation phase, the operator passively stretches the muscle by furthering side-bending movement to the opposite side (4; Fig. **172**).

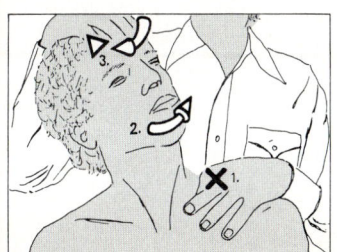
Fig. **171**

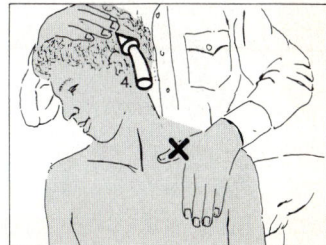
Fig. **172**

Note

- The treatment procedure should be immediately terminated when signs of possible vertebral artery compression develop, such as vertigo, nausea, or spontaneous nystagmus.

Manual Therapy
Iliopsoas Muscle

Treatment

Stretching (NMT 2).

Indication

- Diminished hip extension.
- Soft endfeel due to shortening of the iliopsoas muscle.
- The pain is often diffuse in the inguinal or abdominal region.
- In addition, the erector spinae muscle in the lumbar area is often shortened and the abdominal muscles are quite frequently weakened.

Treatment Procedure

- Patient standing at the end of the examination table.
- The examination table is adjusted to the level of the patient's sacrum.
- The nontreatment leg is maximally flexed at the hip and knee and held up by the patient.
- Under the guidance of the operator, the patient is then reclined onto the examination table. The pelvis is stabilized.
- With the operator providing an equal but opposite resistant force, the patient is requested to contract isometrically the involved iliopsoas muscle for 7–10 seconds (1).
- During the postisometric relaxation phase, the muscle is stretched by increasing hip extension (2; Fig. **173**).

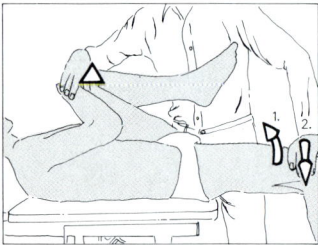

Fig. **173**

Note

- The lumbar lordosis must be reversed during this procedure (support through a neck roll introducing cerebral spine flexion).

Manual Therapy
Rectus femoris Muscle

Treatment

Stretching, NMT 2.

Indication

- Diminished hip flexion with soft endfeel.
- Shortening of the rectus femoris muscle.
- Localized or diffuse thigh pain.

Treatment Procedure

- Patient is prone.
- The operator stabilizes the patient's pelvis with one hand.
- Utilizing passive knee flexion, the hip is extended as far as possible.
- The patient is then requested to contract isometrically the shortened rectus femoris muscle against equal but opposite resistance (1) for approximately 7–10 seconds (Fig. **174a**).
- During the postisometric relaxation phase, the rectoris femoris muscle is stretched further by increasing hip extension (Fig. **174b**).

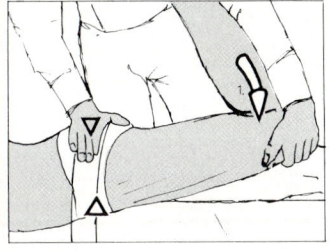

Fig. 174a   Fig. 174b

Note

- This is one of the most frequently shortened muscles.

Manual Therapy
Piriformis Muscle

Treatment

Stretching, NMT 2.

Indication

- With the hip flexed, thigh adduction and external rotation are diminished.
- Soft endfeel.
- The pain can be localized to the buttocks region.
- Pain may also radiate towards the thigh.
- Pain induced with movement which may be localized or projected.
- Localized pain upon palpation of the muscle.

Treatment Procedure

- Patient is supine and flexes the hip to 70°.
- The operator stabilizes the patient's pelvis and then introduces adduction to the thigh to the extreme (barrier) of movement.
- The patient is then requested to contract isometrically the piriform muscle against equal but opposite resistance (1; Fig. **175a**).
- During the postisometric relaxation phase, the shortened piriform muscle is stretched (2) by the operator's further adducting the leg at the hip (Fig. **175b**).

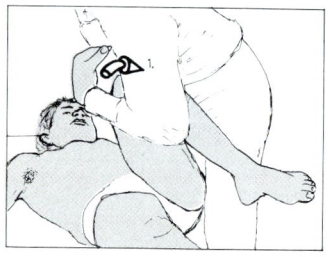
Fig. **175a**

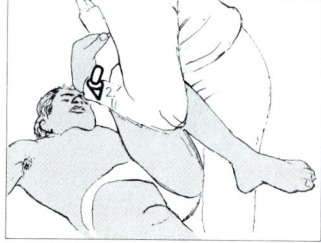
Fig. **175b**

Note

- The possibility of hip joint disease must be excluded.
- Radicular irritation of the sciatic nerve must be differential-diagnostically excluded.

Manual Therapy
Biceps femoris Muscle, Semitendinosus Muscle, Semimembranosus Muscle

Treatment

Stretching, NMT 2.

Indication

- Hip flexion is diminished with the knee extended.
- Soft endfeel with pain at the extreme (barrier) of movement.
- Chronic stretch pain at the posterior thigh.

Treatment Procedure

- Patient is supine.
- The patient's pelvis is fixated against the table with a belt.
- With the patient's knee extended, the operator introduces hip flexion to the barrier (passive flexion).
- The patient is then requested to contract isometrically and against equal but opposite resistance the hamstring muscles (1; Fig. **176**).
- During the postisometric relaxation phase, the muscles are passively stretched by the operator's increasing hip flexion (2).

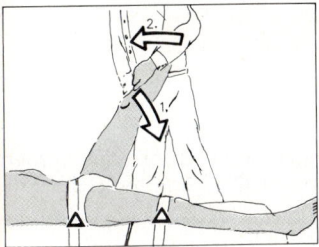

Fig. **176**

Note

- The hamstring muscles are some of the most frequently shortened muscles.

Back School

Aim

Prevention.
- Through:
  a) Improvement of overall physical fitness
  b) Reduction of inappropriate, uneconomical posture and movement patterns; automatic stereotypes need to be altered,
- This can only occur when:
  — the patient can be motivated to become the responsible participant,
  — the patient recognizes and learns about his or her own fitness and abilities as well as limits,
  — the patient enhances his or her consciousness about posture and movements so that he or she can continually evaluate these and eventually correct them as the need arises.
- This requires that both physician and physical therapist
  — cooperate well,
  — have a good knowledge of the field, and
  — invest the necessary time and patience.
- It is not enough
  — just to hand out a few exercises, via pamphlets, or
  — just to inform about ergonomic posture at work.

Content

Overview

This may serve as a recommendation for a back school program to be headed by a physical therapist with 12 lessons, each 50 minutes long:

Lesson 1: Lecture by the Physician
Lesson 2: Muscle Stretching
Lesson 3: Spinal Mobilization 1
Lesson 4: Spinal Mobilization 2
Lesson 5: Strength
Lesson 6: Strength Endurance 1
Lesson 7: Strength Endurance 2
Lesson 8: Coordination 1
Lesson 9: Coordination 2
Lesson 10: Aerobic Endurance 1
Lesson 11: Aerobic Endurance 2
Lesson 12: Encouragement to Actively Participate in Sports

Back School

- Depending on the group's composition, the following factors are considered and individually emphasized:
  - mobility,
  - strength,
  - endurance,
  - coordination.
- Depending on the performance level of the individual group, the exercises can range from easy to difficult, from simple to complex movement patterns.

Participants

- Patients with spinal problems in the subacute to the chronic stage *without* radicular symptomatology.
- The patients must be willing to cooperate and to become a member of a group.
- One of the best ways to determine which patient belongs in which group is to utilize such criteria as mobility and strength. The patient's gender should not be a critical determinant.
- Group size should be kept small, with maximum of 10 members.

Therapist

- The therapist should obtain a good history of the patient's back pain as well as the various activities the patient is involved in at work and in his leisure time.
- A significant motivating factor is the "role model effect" of the therapist; he or she must indentify him- or herself fully with the concept of the back school. The therapist must be able to encourage and stimulate the patient by having a positive outlook him- or herself.
- Authoritative demeanor is a negative learning factor and should be avoided. The willingness to communicate with the patient is very important.

Low Back Pain Program

Lecture by the physician

- Objectives:
  - presentation of theoretical principles
    a) for a better understanding of the overall program and
    b) to help develop an internal understanding and visualization of movement;
  - positive influence on the overall group dynamic process.

Back School

- Content:
  - Anatomy/biomechanics of the spine
  - Pathology
  - Spondylogenic pain
  - Muscular imbalance
  - Posture and movement
  - Information about additional diagnostic procedures, examination techniques, medications, assistive devices, surgical intervention, etc.
  - Discussion
- The theoretical aspects should be presented in a brief but clear manner, utilizing overhead projectors, slides, and a skeleton model for demonstration purposes.

Practical Lessons

- The patient's basic goal is to improve the following factors:
  - Mobility
    a) muscle stretching and
    b) mobilization of the spine and peripheral joints
  - Strength and strength endurance
  - Coordination
  - Endurance

This will then lead to better posture and movement as well as increased awareness of what is appropriate movement.

Mobility

- Muscle stretching:

  Shortened tonic muscles inhibit their phasic antagonists as well as synergistic muscles, allowing muscular imbalance to develop.
  If this muscular imbalance can be positively influenced, the musculoskeletal system and the spine can react to other outside challenges more appropriately.

- *Exercise Program*

  Stretching, passive static and active static:
  - Hamstring muscles
  - Lumbar back extensors
  - Deep gluteal muscles
  - Hip flexors
  - Adductors
  - Calf muscles
  - Neck and chest muscles

Back School

- *Note*
  - The selection of the starting position for the individual muscles should be individualized for the requirements of a particular group of participants.
  - The exercises must be explained clearly, and the patient's performance should be corrected whenever necessary.
  - The stretching program should also be performed at home on a regular basis.

- *Mobilization*
  The goal of mobilization is to improve mobility in the various spinal segments and regions.

- *Exercise Program*
  Active mobilization, lumbar spine/pelvis,
  thoracic spine/thorax,
  cervical spine/shoulder girdle,
  starting from the simple and progressing to the more difficult starting positions. Relationships between movement in the pelvis, legs, arms, and spine should be addressed specifically and repeatedly emphasized.

- *Note*
  These exercise should also help in the activities of daily life, where they may serve to decrease pain so as to improve the musculoskeletal system's reaction to outside forces and to help in relaxation as well.

Strength/Strength Endurance

The goal is to train for strength in those muscles that stabilize the thrunk, required by the activities of daily life.

- *Exercise Program*
  Strengthening, Dynamic—slow:
  - Straight and oblique abdominal muscles
  - Gluteal muscles (gluteus maximum, medius, and minimis muscles)
  - Shoulder blade fixator muscles
  - Thoracic spine extensor muscles

- *Note*
  - Correct execution of these exercises is important; tonic synergy patterns must be eliminated, assuring correct movement sequences as well as appropriate breathing techniques.
  - In order to assure appropriate results with these techniques, the patient's limits and program must be determined.
  - Appropriate instruction must be given for home training exercises.

Back School

Coordination

Good motor coordination can only occur when there is a harmonious, effective, and economical interplay between movements.

- *Exercise Program*
  Of use are exercise on nonstationary surfaces (ball), exercises for lower extremity movement, and exercises for upper extremity involvement.

Endurance

While in the back school, the participant should be stimulated to also get involved in aerobic endurance training such as swimming, bicycle riding, jogging, and cross-country skiing.
The person should be motivated to improve present physical stamina by actively participating in a program.

- *Exercise Program*
  - working on an economical running technique
  - Pulse measurements (180 minus patient's age)
  - Appropriate breathing techniques
  - Development of a training program (stretching, regeneration, loading forces, etc.)

Important Features That Should Be Included in Each Lesson

- Discussion: questions should be answered.
- "Warming up" to improve stretchability of the tissues. As the starting point for endurance training, the intensity of the warming-up period progresses from one lesson to the next.
- The patient must be instructed to breath appropriately.
- Relaxation and certain other positions that would decrease stress and load on the musculoskeletal system must be integrated into the patient's daily routines.
- Activities of daily living: Appropriate lying and sitting, standing and bending or stooping, lifting and carrying.
- Ergonomics in the workplace and economical movement patterns. This should not be a separate portion, but rather integrated into each lesson.
- Alternating static and dynamic influences; the participant in a group should become aware of these changes and integrate them appropriately into his activities of daily life.
- Repetition; continued and regular repetition is of the utmost importance and the home program must be re-evaluated from time to time.
- The exercise group should be challenging but not disappointing to the patient, as this is a good way of learning about one's individual abilities.
- Last, but not least, this program should be fun and should motivate the participant to pick up other training methods and exercises that he or she can perform on his or her own and on a regular basis.

References

Dvorak J. Funktionelle Anatomie der oberen Halswirbelsäule unter besonderer Berücksichtigung des Bandapparates. In: Wolff H.D., ed. Die Sonderstellung der Kopfgelenke. Berlin: Springer, 1988: 19–46.

Dvorak J., Panjabi M. Functional anatomy of the alar ligaments. Spine 1987; 12:2:183–8.

Dvorak J., Panjabi M., Gerber M., Wichmann W. CT-functional diagnostics of the rotatory instability of upper cervical spine. Spine 1987; 12:3:197–205.

Dvorak J., Froehlich D., Penning L. Functional radiographic diagnosis of the cervical spine. Spine 1988; 13:748–55.

Fassbender H.G. Der rheumatische Schmerz. MW 1980; 31:36:1263–67.

Fielding J.W. Cineroentgenography of the normal cervical spine. JBJS 1957; 39A:6:1280–8.

Janda V. Muskelfunktionsdiagnostik. Leuven: Fisher, 1979.

Kapandji A. The physiology of joints: the trunk and vertebral column. London: Churchill-Livingstone, 1974.

Knese K. Kopfhaltung und Kopfbewegung des Menschen. Z Anat Entwickl Gesch 1947/50; 114;67–87.

Lewit K. Manuelle Medizin im Rahmen der medizinischen Rehabilitation. 5th ed. München: Urban & Schwarzenberg, 1987.

Rickenbacher J., Landolt A.M., Theiler K. Rücken: Praktische Anatomie. 1st ed. Heidelberg: Springer, 1982:408. (Lanz T., Wachsmuth W., ed. Praktische Anatomie; vol 7).

Sutter M. Versuch einer Wesensbestimmung pseudoradikulärer Syndrome. Schweiz Rundsch Med Prax 1974; 63:842–848.

White A., Panjabi P. Clinical biomechanics of the spine. 2nd ed. Philadelphia: Lippincott, 1990.

Index

A
Abdominal muscles, strength and endurance testing, 102–103
Ankle joint *see* Foot
Atlantoaxial joint
  axes of movement, 12
  transected, 13
  see also Cervical spine
Atlanto–occipital joint
  alar ligaments, 14–15
  axes of movement, 12
  ligamentous apparatus, 14
  ranges of movement, 11
  see also Cervical spine
Atlas vertebra
  palpation of the transverse process, 40–41
  see also Cervical spine

B
Back school
  coordination program, 178
  endurance program, 178
  low back pain program, content and practical lesson, 175–176
  mobility, exercise program, 137, 176–177
  participants, 175
  program content, 174
    principles, 178
  strength/endurance program, 177
  therapist, 175
Biceps femoris muscle
  length testing, 100–101
  stretching, NMT-2, 173
Biomechanics of the spine, 1–25
  primary axes, 9, 10

C
Calf, phasic/tonic muscles, 5
Cervical spine
  C0–C1
    flexion and extension, 30
    mobilization without impulse, flexion and extension, 138
    zones of irritation, 106
  C0–C3
    anatomic relationships and motion, 11–14
    axial rotation, 31
    biomechanics, 11–15
    end rotation of the axis, 40–41
    forced rotation of the axis, 39–40
    mobilization without impulse, axial traction, 139
    provocative testing, 33
  C1–C2
    axial rotation, 32
    mobilization utilizing postisometric relaxation of antagonists, 140
  C2–C6
    mobilization with impulse, and rotation, 142
    mobilization with impulse, rotation restriction, 141, 145
  C2–C7
    mobilization utilizing postisometric relaxation of antagonists, 143–144
    provocative testing, 108–109
    zones of irritation, 107–109
  C3–C6, axial rotation, 45
  C3–C7
    anatomic relationships and motion, 14–17
    axial rotation, 13, 15, 16
    biomechanics, 15–18
    facet joints and axes of movement, 15
    segmental arches of movement, 16
    vertebral artery, 17
  cervicothoracic junction
    axial rotation, 38, 44
    flexion and extension, 36, 42
    mobilization with impulse, and rotation, 146
    mobilization with impulse, side-bending restriction, 147
    rotation with extension, 34–35
    side-bending, 37, 43
  De Kleijn hanging test, 18
  radiologic diagnosis, 117–118
  reclination test, 17
  vertebral artery *see* Vertebral artery
Craniocervical junction *see* Atlanto–occipital joint

D
De Kleijn hanging test, cervical spine, 18
Diskopathies, root irritation, 53–55, 101
Dizziness *see* Vertigo

Index

E
Elbow
  pronation and supination, motion testing, 66
  radiohumeral joint, traction and gliding movement, 68
  radioulnar joint, translatory motion testing, 67
Enkephalins
  production by spinal cord, 24
  release from joints in dysfunctional positions, 25
Erector spinae muscles, length testing, 92–93

F
Foot
  ankle joint, translatory movement
    calcaneal–cuboid joint, 81
    gliding movement, 78
    talonavicular joint, 79
    talus and cuneiform bones, 80
  phasic/tonic muscles, 5
  tarsometatarsal joint, translatory movement testing, 82

G
Gluteus maximus muscle, strength testing, 104
Gluteus medius muscle, strength testing, 105

H
Hamstrings
  biceps femoris muscle
    length testing, 100–101
    stretching, NMT-2, 173
  semimembranosus muscle
    length testing, 100–101
    stretching, NMT-2, 173
  semitendinosus muscle
    length testing, 100–101
    stretching, NMT-2, 173
Hand
  interphalangeal joints, translation testing, 73
  metacarpal joints, translatory gliding movement, 72
  metacarpophalangeal joints, translation testing, 73
  primary carpals, palpation and functional examination, 71
  proximal carpals, palpation and angular movement, 70
  radiocarpal joint, translatory movement, 69
Home exercise program *see* Back school
5-Hydroxytryptamine, action, 23

I
Iliac spine, posterior superior, sacroiliac joint nutation, 57–58
Iliolumbar ligament, provocative testing, 55
Iliopsoas muscle, stretching, NMT-2, 170
Ilium *see* Sacroiliac joint
Intervertebral joints
  innervation, 23–24
  neurophysiology, 22–24

J
Joints, neurophysiology, 22–24

K
Kibler skin fold, 27
Knee joints
  axial traction, axial rotation, anterior and posterior translation, 75–76
  femoropatellar gliding, 74
  proximal tibiofibular joints, 77

L
Lasgue sign
  pseudo-Lasgue sign, 101
  reversed, 99
Levator scapulae muscle
  length testing, 86–87
  stretching, NMT-2, 168
Longissimus lumborum muscles, length testing, 92–93
Lumbar spine
  axial rotation, 53
  biomechanics, 18–19
  diskopathies, 53–55
  facet joints and axes of movement, 19, 19
  facet syndrome, 51
  flexion and extension, 51
  lower, provocative testing of the iliolumbar ligament, 55
  mobilization with impulse flexion and extension, 160

Index

Lumbar spine mobilization with impulse
  rotation, 157–159
  mobilization without impulse NMT-2, rotation, 156
  rotation, 155
  radiologic diagnosis, 121–127
    AP views, 121, 123
    lateral views, 124–127
  side-bending, 52
  spondylarthrosis, 51, 53
  spondylolisthesis, 55
  springing test, 54
  traction spurs (marks), 126–127
  zones of irritation, 113–114
Lumbosacral junction, pelvic torsion, 125
Lunate bone, palpation and functional examination, 70–71

M

Manual therapy
  contraindications, 130
  extremity joints, 133
  indications, 128–129
  principles, 131
  vertebral column, mobilization without/with impulse, 132–133
  see also specific joints and regions
Mechanoreceptors, 22
Meniscoid, anatomic arrangement, 22–23
Muscle *see* Skeletal muscle
Myosis
  etiology, 7
  pathology, 8
Myotendinosis
  defined, 4
  pathology, 8
  spondylogenic reflex syndrome, 29
Myotenone
  defined, 8
  types, 9

N

Nausea and dizziness *see* Vertigo
Neuromuscular therapy
  mobilization
    direct muscle force of agonists, 134
    postisometric relaxation of antagonists, 134–136
    reciprocal inhibition of the antagonists, 136
NMT *see* Neuromuscular therapy
Nociceptors, 22–23

O

Occiput *see* Atlanto–occipital joint
Opioids, naturally produced *see* Enkephalins

P

Paravertebral muscles
  anatomic relationships, 1
  conflict situation, 2–3
Patrick–Faber test, sacroiliac joints, 59
Pectoralis major muscle
  length testing, 83
  stretching, NMT-2, 166
Pelvic girdle
  anatomic arrangement and function, 19–21
  arch-type (high assimilation), 125
  flat-type, 125
  functional unit, 19
  normal (block) pelvis, 125
  pelvic torsion, 122, 125
  radiologic diagnosis, 121–122
  sacroiliac joint
    anatomic arrangement and function, 19–21
    see also Sacroiliac joint
  symphysis, shearing forces, 19–22
  and thigh, phasic/tonic muscles, 5
Piriform muscle
  length testing, 94–95
  stretching, NMT-2, 172
Pisiform bone, palpation and functional examination, 70–71
Postural muscles
  fast/slow twitch fibers, 3
  functional pathology, 3
  overview, 6
PSIS *see* Iliac spine, posterior superior
Psoas major muscle, length testing, 96–97

R

Radiologic diagnosis, 117–127
  cervical spine, 117–118
  lumbar spine, 121–127

pelvic girdle, 121–122
sacroiliac joint, 122–123
thoracic spine, 119–120
Reclination test, cervical spine, 17
Rectus femoris muscle
  length testing, 98–99
  stretching, NMT-2, 171
Rheumatism, noninflammatory soft-tissue
  etiology, 7
  pathology, 8
Ribs
  rib I
    "elevated first rib," 91
    mobilization without impulse, 152
    passive motion testing, 49
  ribs III to XII, respiratory excursion of the individual ribs, 50
  ribs III–X, mobilization with impulse, 154
  ribs VI–XII, mobilization without impulse, 153
  scalene muscles, length testing, 90–91
  zones of irritation, 112
  see also Thoracic spine

S

Sacroiliac joint
  anatomic arrangement, 19–21
  body posture and effects, 21
  degenerative change, 20
  mobilization with impulse, 163, 164, 165
  mobilization without impulse, NMT-1 162
    anterior motion restriction (ventralization), 161
  "nutation" (nodding) movement, 21
    spine and standing flexion tests, 56–57
  passive motion test, 58
  Patrick–Faber test, 59
  pelvic girdle, zones of irritation, 115–116
  radiologic diagnosis, 122–123
  sacral suspension, 20
Scalene muscles, length testing, 90–91
Scalenus anticus syndrome, 49

Scaphoid bone, palpation and functional examination, 70–71
Scapula *see* Levator scapulae muscle; Shoulder girdle
Scoliosis, compensatory, in acute disk herniation, 93
Semitendinosus muscle, stretching, NMT-2, 173
Serotonin *see* 5-Hydroxytryptamine
Shoulder girdle
  acromioclavicular joint, translatory motion testing, 61
  glenohumeral joint
    anterior gliding, 65
    axial traction, 62
    inferior gliding, 63
    superior gliding, 64
  phasic/tonic muscles, 5
  sternoclavicular joint, 60
Skeletal muscles
  fast/slow twitch fibers compared, 4
  functional pathology, 3
  neuromuscular therapy, 134–136
  palpation, 27–28, 27–29
  phasic/tonic muscles, 4, 5
  spondylogenic reflex syndrome, 29
  vertebral column, rotation and coupling pattern, 9, 10, 11
  zones of irritation, 28–29
Skin-rolling test, 27
Spina bifida occulta, 124
Spine *see* Vertebral column
Spondylogenic reflex syndrome, 29
Sternocleidomastoid muscle
  length testing, 88–89
  stretching, NMT-2, 169

T

Talocrural joint *see* Foot, ankle joint
Tendinoses, types, 8
Thigh/pelvic girdle, phasic/tonic muscles, 5
Thoracic outlet syndrome, 91
Thoracic spine
  biomechanics, 18
  facet joints and axes of movement, 18
  gross motion testing, 19

Thoracic spine
  radiologic diagnosis, 119–120
  T1–T12
    flexion and extension, 46
    side-bending, 47
    zones of irritation, 110–111
  T3–L1, axial rotation, 48
  T3–T10
    mobilization with impulse, 148, 149
    mobilization without impulse, rotation, 150
  T6–T12, mobilization with impulse, rotation, 151
  see also Ribs
Traction spurs (marks), lumbar spine, 126–127
Trapezius muscle
  length testing, 84–85
  stretching, NMT-2, 167
Triquetrum, palpation and functional examination, 70–71
Trunk, phasic/tonic muscles, 5

V

Ventralization maneuver, 116, 161
Vertebrae
  model for receptor activity, correct/incorrect position, 25
  segmental dysfunction, 25–26
  vertebral unit (motion segment), 10

Vertebral artery
  compression see Vertigo
  course, 17
  provocative testing of C0–C3, 33
  reclination test, 17
Vertebral column
  anatomy and biomechanics, 1–25
  back school, home exercise program, 137, 172–178
  biomechanics, 1–25
  examination, 26
    see also specific regions
  manual therapy, mobilization without/with impulse, 132–133
  paravertebral muscles, 1–3
  paravertebral palpation of the skin, 26–27
  see also Cervical spine; Lumbar spine; Pelvic girdle; Thoracic spine;
Vertigo, caused by compression of vertebral artery, 33, 35, 89, 169

W

Wrist see Hand

Z

Zones of irritation, 106–116
  defined, 28